Serious Games in Physical Rehabilitation

Bruno Bonnechère

Serious Games in Physical Rehabilitation

From Theory to Practice

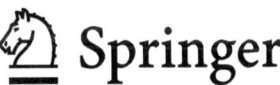 Springer

Bruno Bonnechère
Laboratory of Anatomy
Biomechanics and Organogenesis
Université Libre de Bruxelles
Brussels, Belgium

Department of Electronic and Informatics - ETRO
Vrije Universiteit Brussel, Brussels, Belgium imec
Leuven, Belgium

ISBN 978-3-319-66121-6   ISBN 978-3-319-66122-3   (eBook)
https://doi.org/10.1007/978-3-319-66122-3

Library of Congress Control Number: 2017956924

Printed on acid-free paper

This Springer imprint is published by Springer Nature
The registered company is Springer International Publishing AG
The registered company address is: Gewerbestrasse 11, 6330 Cham, Switzerland

Preface

At first sight, for an uninformed reader, the title of this book must seem a bit unusual. Actually, there may be a double astonishment.

The first one is this term *serious* attached to game: how can games be serious since they are associated, for most people, with pleasure and fun? This first point is nevertheless not too difficult to clarify since lots of games are serious (e.g., chess, Go) and/or used to develop skills (e.g., management, reflection).

Actually, the title of this book should have been the use of serious *video* games in physical rehabilitation. Indeed, in the last sixty years, video games have been developed and are becoming every day more and more popular within the population. While traditional games are accepted by most people and recognized as beneficial the use of video games is more problematic. The most frequent criticisms about video games are that they would be responsible for an increase in violence, decrease in social contacts, and would turn the players more sedentary.

This leads to the second contradiction of the title of this book: video games and physical therapy. Should not rehabilitation medicine be something serious and not something fun?

The aim of this book is therefore to demonstrate that video games can indeed be serious and used, successfully, in rehabilitation.

The transition of gaming consoles from the living room to the hospital and the clinic is not that obvious and is far away from the classical development of medical devices.

The typical stages of development and integration of new medical devices are request from the clinics (need), team of researchers (engineers, doctors, etc.) working on a prototype, and then several interactions between clinics and the research to get the final product. This is the classic translation between research and clinics. Whether or not this product needs to be validated before being used in clinics is debatable for medical devices whereas the questions about efficacy, effectiveness, and safety are, naturally, not an option for drugs.

The integration of serious games within the rehabilitation is totally different: the products have been designed and developed for fun and entertainment and then some clinicians seeing a possible clinical interest tried to use the games with their patients. It is only later on that researchers and developers have had interest for this field and tried to develop specific games for rehabilitation, first based on existing gaming device and then by developing specific devices too.

Both development of new medical devices and rehabilitation medicine being highly multidisciplinary, this book has thus to be as broad and comprehensive as possible.

In order to understand how video games could be used in clinics, it is important to have a clear view of the current available technologies and what are the next expected improvements.

As serious as they can be, serious games are still games, we will see how the traditional games have been developed since ages and can be used for rehabilitation, and then of course the rise of video games for entertainment and then in the healthcare domain.

The most important part of this book is the discussion about the clinical efficacy and safety of such kind of new intervention for various pathologies and how to integrate serious games within the conventional rehabilitation.

More than ever, in the global context of reducing healthcare costs, medical devices must be validated in clinics in order to have a chance to be reimbursed; therefore well-designed and controlled randomized clinical trial should be conducted in this field, and an example is provided in this book.

Some people often forget that the last step of the translational process between research and patient is…business! Therefore in the last part of this book we will present some business aspects focusing on innovation and novelty, the two key elements to develop a sustainable business.

Brussels, Belgium   Bruno Bonnechère

Contents

The Technology

"Let's go invent tomorrow instead of worrying about what happened yesterday."

– Steve Jobs

1.1 The Computers

Without computers anything of this would be possible! The growth of the computational power of modern computers is exponential implying continuously increasing progress in the gaming industry as well. The first computer—the ENIAC (Electronic Numerical Integrator and Computer)—has been built in 1946 and occupied a full room for a weight of 30 Tons. The computer games evolved from early days of computers and forked from research applications like simulations and demonstrations developed to entertain the public. In 70 years, the computational power has been drastically increasing and we moved from text-based games to realistic virtual and immersive environments. However, considering the exponential growth, in a few decades will people look at the current games the same way as we look to the "Pong" or the "Pacman." In parallel to this growth, the size and the price of the technology is decreasing at the same rate.

The first microprocessor was built in 1971; since that date the power of processors have been increasing exponentially. Moore's law stipulated that the power of computer is doubled every 18 months since every innovation boosts the creation of new products (Moore 1965).

The increase of power calculation allowed the development of applications requiring a lot of computational power such as visual graphics, particularly important for the development of video games.

1.2   The Graphical (R)evolution

The evolution of computer graphics can be seen more easily than the computational power. The first video games were developed from the 1950s and evolved mainly from research/instructional programs, simulations, and demonstrators. They were mostly text based shaping its appearance to remind simple geometrical objects[1]. The need for visualization required for many applications created the basis for 2D graphics technology. Associated to this technology's evolution, the scenario and the complexity of the games never stopped and in the modern games the player is literally immersed in a gaming environment which looks closer to the reality. There are plenty of serious games that are developed and used in various fields (e.g., to increase workers' safety by simulating of various situations, to increase performance in sports (e.g., driving simulation), to practice safely prior being in real situation (e.g., flight simulator training, etc.)).

1.3   The Three-Dimensional Environment

The 3D computer graphics, pioneered by William Fetter, put extra demand on the computational resources creating a gap of few decades between the first computers and consumer 3D applications. Although the first publicly available 3D graphics software and games is from the 1970s, the popularity rose in 1990s and with the new millennia. Wide public could observe the high-quality 3D animations with series of successful blog buster movies (Tron, Terminator 2, Jurassic Park, Toy Story, Avatar, etc.). However, the industry that drives and demonstrates the evolution of 3D technologies the most is video gaming industry. The graphics has evolved from games that used only a few simple primitives (e.g., lines in the game Battlezone) through richer graphics (e.g., Wolfenstein 3D) to realistic environments with procedurally generated content and advanced artificial intelligence (e.g., The Elder Scrolls IV: Oblivion). The power to render realistic environments is now embedded into many households in the form of a game console or an entertainment system (e.g., MS Xbox One, Sony PlayStation 4). The upcoming trend is involving immersive 3D in the form of virtual reality, often based on a stereoscopic image requiring headset or glasses. Increased immersion is often achieved by including natural interactions (for humans) between humans and computer. This involves free movement of the player's body tracking allowing new and unconventional kinds of interactions.

Majority of the modern computer games use advanced 3D systems (LaViola 2008), and it is expected that in the near future this technology will be adopted within our daily activities including health-related applications. Scientists from around the world are working on many examples, e.g., for people with depth perception impairment or other cognitive and physical disabilities.

---

[1] For example, the Pong game consists of two lines and a point.

A lot of the low-cost gaming devices have already spawned completely new research tracks. Gaming input devices, often resemble medically used devices. Open the potential for everyday use. For instance, MS Kinect allows real-time body tracking, the Wii balance board tracking center of the pressure, but also smart phones—equipped by IMU—tracking orientation and positional information of the device. Also, novel output devices offer potential changes in perception on tap. For instance, the Oculus Rift™ is a pioneering device, a headset using virtual reality, that allows (along an immersive experience) rapid changes in environment at rate that would not be possible in the physical world.

Scientists and researchers are adopting these disruptive technologies in plenty of research projects and clinical application. By using these devices allowing complete immersion of the patients, they allow them to experience various situations that could be hardly achieved during traditional treatment or rehabilitation exercises. Therefore, some other neuronal circuits and zones of the brain can be trained.

1.4 The Internet

The development and the generalization of high-speed Internet connection had changed the traditional games to a tool for social interaction. With the development of smartphones and mobile broadband connection people can interact not only in the real-time but also on the go. This network enables interconnect mobile devices with remote servers and server farms with much performant machines—distributing the high computational demand in the mobile devices. Therefore, a new approach to game development emerges where most of the computation can be done on the cloud.

Offloading the mobile devices to the cloud helps the game development studios establish a new business model where the game is offered as a service rather than of-the-shelf package. Another consequence is that the cloud empowers even broader social interactions among the players. The Massively Multiplayer Online Game (MMOG) and the Massively Multiplayer Online Role-Playing Games (MMORPG) are now one of the keystones in the video games industry. The revenue generated by MMOG and MMORPG never ceased to increase since introduced to the market in the 1990s. In 2012, the revenue for games industries was about 21 billion \$[2]; the part for MMOG and MMORPG is approximately 25%. In 2014, the numbers were 25.3 billion \$ with 27% for online games[3].

Of course, serious games specifically developed for patients currently do not reach the same levels but we can observe the same trends in the serious games focused on health. The MMOG have even the potential to engage the disabled patients by supporting interactions with their healthy counterparts within a single environment. Through the anonymity of the Internet, this may offer a new

---

[2] http://www.theesa.com/facts/pdfs/ESA_EF_2013.pdf
[3] The Video Gaming Industry Outlook

socializing tool transparent in terms of the game, but still containing the serious aspects of the therapy.

1.5   The Commercial Video Games

Commercial video games have significantly evolved over the last decades to one of the biggest markets (generated almost $100 billion in revenues in 2016 globally[4]) in the entertainment industry with the accelerating annual growth of 8.5%. However, as the world becomes more connected and more of our activities are performed on mobile devices, some experts predict decline in sales of gaming consoles and game-purposed computers. The manufacturers of the gaming hardware therefore tend to concentrate their focus on the most compelling gaming experience and disruptive innovations. For instance, game controllers (Nintendo Wii Fit™, Microsoft Xbox Kinect™, Sony Play Station™, etc.) change the traditional passive video gameplay (i.e., controlling the game with mouse or a keyboard) to an active experience where the players are required to move in order to interact with games.

The new trends in game controllers is not only transforming the way the games are played, but it also led scientists to focus their attention on these devices due to their potential in clinical and/or scientific applications. Businesses have already started to focus on providing clinically relevant data collected from these devices. Therefore, in the next sections we are going to briefly present the game consoles coming with novel controllers that gained popularity in motion analysis and physical therapy in particular. We also describe our expectations on how these controllers could be, or already are, used for health-related applications mainly in physical rehabilitation.

1.5.1   From Games to Sciences?

This new trend of games controlling and controllers has not only completely modified the way of playing video games, but also led scientists to focus on these new devices for future potential clinical and/or scientific applications. Indeed, we are going to see that some game controllers present interesting characteristics similar to the devices that are used to perform motion analysis in clinics. Therefore in the next subchapters, we are going to present game consoles and controllers from a gaming point of view and then describe how these controllers could be used, or are already used, for other applications such as motion analysis, patients evaluation, and follow-up or rehabilitation.

---

[4] https://newzoo.com/insights/articles/global-games-market-reaches-99-6-billion-2016-mobile-generating-37/

1.5.2   Nintendo Wii

1.5.2.1 The Gaming Aspects

The Nintendo Wii is one of the first video game consoles using motion of the human body and novel controllers that were successfully adopted by the mass market. This console has been released on November 2006 and turned out to be a success with immediate worldwide sales. Unlike previous consoles, the games have been controlled by the Wii remote controller which detects motions of the players in three dimensions using inertial measurement sensors. In July 2007, the Wii Balance Board (WBB), a force plate that measures center of pressure, was released allowing players to control the games using center of pressure displacement. Most of the games using these controllers focus on fitness-related games, body movement, and burn calories of the player.

1.5.2.2 The Scientific Aspects

The evaluation of balance and postural control is an important field in various domains such as health (e.g., preventions of falls in elderly people), rehabilitation (e.g., balance training after stroke), and sports (e.g., to increase athlete's performance or decrease injuries' risk). Despite this potential huge field of application, it appears that balance assessment using a force plate (FP) (i.e., during quantitative functional evaluation) in laboratory is not as used as it should be in clinics for patients' evaluation or follow-up. Despite this, the measurement of the center of pressure (CP) using FP is considered as gold standard to assess balance (Haas and Burden 2000). This is probably due to the fact that FPs are, most of the time, not transportable due to their embedment in the laboratory floor. Their relatively high price is also blocking their widespread use outside the laboratory. Access to this kind of tool is therefore limited and does not allow regular measurement for patient follow-up or evaluation of a treatment if a specially equipped laboratory is not available.

In daily clinics, evaluation of balance is performed using scales such as the qualitative Berg Balance Scale. Despite the fact that these scales have been validated for various neurological conditions, they are not sensitive enough to detect small clinically relevant changes (Blum and Korner-Bitensky 2008). There is thus a need in clinics for portable, easy-to-use, and cost-effective quantitative balance assessment tools. The Wii Balance Board™ meets the above criteria. But before being used in clinics such kind of devices must, of course, go through a strict validation process. Several works have been done to validate the WBB: estimation of CP path length during standing (Clark et al. 2010, Huurnink et al. 2013) and force estimation (Bartlett et al. 2014). In clinics, the WBB has been used to assess patients suffering from various diseases such as Parkinson's disease (Holmes et al. 2013) or other conditions as, for instance, anterior cruciate ligament injuries (Howells et al. 2013), and with elderly patients (Young et al. 2011, Koslucher et al. 2012).

1.5.3   Sony PlayStation

1.5.3.1 The Gaming Aspects

This console is mainly used with traditional gamepad. However, two other components can be used to control the games. The PlayStation eye toy is a digital camera able to detect the player and recognize the motion to allow players to interact with the games. The other one is the PlayStation move, a motion-sensing game controller using inertial sensor (similar system as the Nintendo Wii Remote controller). Despite the existence of these two controllers, most of the games are being played with the gamepad.

1.5.3.2 The Scientific Aspects

To our best knowledge, there is currently no published work about the use of neither the eye toy nor the move controller for performing motion analysis. By cons as discussed in the chapter Serious Games in Rehabilitation, these devices are used in rehabilitation.

1.5.4   Microsoft Xbox Kinect

1.5.4.1 The Gaming Aspects

The release of the MS Kinect in November 2010 marked another milestone in the new direction. In contrast to Nintendo Wii, which uses direct measurements and physical interaction with the controller; the Kinect can track the human body on distance. It tracks a simplified skeleton of the human body from a stream of depth map data[5]. Since the Kinect controller tracks the pose of the player, it allows greater variations of possible controls (e.g., various body gestures) and could help to evaluate the correctness of the performed motion or exercises. The measurements of distance provide better immersion effect and essentially make the controller out of the human body.

1.5.4.2 The Scientific Aspects

The release of the Kinect produced the same enthusiasm among the scientific community as that of the Balance Board. This cost-effective and portable device combines a regular color camera with a depth camera (consisting of an infrared laser projector and an infrared camera) and built-in software to detect a simple skeleton, composed by 20 points representing the major joints of the body.

This model is used to track motions of the players during the games, based on advanced pattern recognition methods.

3D motion analysis using Marker Based Systems (MBS), optoelectronic devices, is considered as Gold Standard for clinical motion analysis even if several issues have been previously raised and discussed in the literature. Such kind of systems are

---

[5]A depth map is a matrix of measurements where each element corresponds to a distance measurement between a camera an object at corresponding location (a.k.a. depth image).

composed of several infrared cameras that tracked simultaneously 3D position of markers glued on the subjects. Positions and trajectories are then reconstructed, thanks to information collected by the cameras.

Accessibility of MBS is an issue due to the costs of such systems, and therefore only specialized centers can afford them. Furthermore, marker placement [i.e., time consuming and potential source of error (Della Croce et al. 2005)] and skin displacement during motion (Leardini et al. 2005) are two recognized problems within the MBS field. The Kinect sensor is a cost-effective and portable MLS device that seems to offer interesting new perspectives for functional analysis and patient assessment. There are plenty of studies that have been conducted in order to test the possibility of the Kinect for motion analysis first with healthy subjects then with patients. Some studies have investigated the precision of the Kinect to detect volume and distance (Dutta 2012), to assess postural control in static (Clark et al. 2012) and in dynamic conditions (Yeung et al. 2014), to assess range of motion for simple planar motions (Bonnechère et al. 2014), for upper limb evaluation to assess reachable workspace on healthy subjects (Kurillo et al. 2013) and on patients suffering from facioscapulohumeral muscular dystrophy (Han et al. 2015), to assess head's posture (Oh et al. 2014), arm movement speed (Elgendi et al. 2014), gait analysis (Pfister et al. 2014), and to track full body motions during serious games exercises (van Diest et al. 2014).

In 2014, a second version of the Kinect sensor was released; gesture recognition and motion tracking were improved with the new generation of sensor (Pagliari and Pinto, 2015).

1.5.5   Other Devices

1.5.5.1 Leap Motion

The Leap Motion Controller is a small sensor equipped with two cameras. This device is mainly used for hand and finger gesture recognition and is used to perform manual task on the computer (e.g., pinch-to-zoom, drawing, or manipulating 3D data visualizations).

Considering the current limitations of the Nintendo Wii remote controller and the Kinect sensor for wrist and finger displacement, the Leap Motion Controller could be the ideal solution to track and train dexterity and fine motor function of the upper limb.

1.5.5.2 Oculus Rift

The Oculus Rift was the first virtual reality headset available in the commerce (for nonprofessional user). The headset integrated an OLED display, headphones for 3D sounds, and gyroscope to detect the position of the head and to adjust the environment accordingly.

A lot of research is currently being conducted using the Oculus Rift, and other kinds of headset, mainly in the domain of phobia or in case of post-traumatic stress disorders.

1.5.5.3 HTC Vive

HTC Vive is a virtual reality head-mounted display and two wireless handheld controllers. This system allows the user to navigate naturally (walk, move objects, etc.), communicate, and experience immersive virtual environments.

This kind of device potentially combining virtual reality immersion and motor rehabilitation paves the way for enormous innovation in physical, and cognitive, rehabilitation.

References

Bartlett HL, Ting LH, Bingham JT. Accuracy of force and center of pressure measures of the Wii balance board. Gait Posture. 2014;39(1):224–8.

Blum L, Korner-Bitensky N. Usefulness of the Berg balance scale in stroke rehabilitation: a systematic review. Phys Ther. 2008;88(5):559–66.

Bonnechère B, Jansen B, Salvia P, Bouzahouene H, Omelina L, Moiseev F, Sholukha V, Cornelis J, Rooze M, Van Sint Jan S. Validity and reliability of the Kinect within functional assessment activities: comparison with standard stereophotogrammetry. Gait Posture. 2014;39(1):593–8.

Clark RA, Bryant AL, Pua Y, McCrory P, Bennell K, Hunt M. Validity and reliability of the Nintendo Wii balance board for assessment of standing balance. Gait Posture. 2010;31(3):307–10.

Clark RA, Pua YH, Fortin K, Ritchie C, Webster KE, Denehy L, Bryant AL. Validity of the Microsoft Kinect for assessment of postural control. Gait Posture. 2012;36(3):372–7.

Della Croce U, Leardini A, Chiari L, Cappozzo A. Human movement analysis using stereophotogrammetry. Part 4: assessment of anatomical landmark misplacement and its effects on joint kinematics. Gait Posture. 2005;21(2):226–37.

van Diest M, Stegenga J, Wörtche HJ, Postema K, Verkerke GJ, Lamoth CJ. Suitability of Kinect for measuring whole body movement patterns during exergaming. J Biomech. 2014;47(12):2925–32.

Dutta T. Evaluation of the KinectTM sensor for 3-D kinematic measurement in the workplace. Appl Ergon. 2012;43(4):645–9.

Elgendi M, Picon F, Magnenat-Thalmann N, Abbott D. Arm movement speed assessment via a Kinect camera: a preliminary study in healthy subjects. Biomed Eng Online. 2014;13:88.

Haas BM, Burden AM. Validity of weight distribution and sway measurements of the balance performance monitor. Physiother Res Int. 2000;5(1):19–32.

Han JJ, Kurillo G, Abresch RT, de Bie E, Nicorici A, Bajcsy R. Reachable workspace in facioscapulohumeral muscular dystrophy (FSHD) by Kinect. Muscle Nerve. 2015;51(2):168–75.

Holmes JD, Jenkins ME, Johnson AM, Hunt MA, Clark RA. Validity of the Nintendo Wii® balance board for the assessment of standing balance in Parkinson's disease. Clin Rehabil. 2013;27(4):361–6.

Howells BE, Clark RA, Ardern CL, Bryant AL, Feller JA, Whitehead TS, Webster KE. The assessment of postural control and the influence of a secondary task in people with anterior cruciate ligament reconstructed knees using a Nintendo Wii balance board. Br J Sports Med. 2013;47(14):914–9.

Huurnink A, Fransz DP, Kingma I, van Dieën JH. Comparison of a laboratory grade force platform with a Nintendo Wii balance board on measurement of postural control in single-leg stance balance tasks. J Biomech. 2013;46(7):1392–5.

Koslucher F, Wade MG, Nelson B, Lim K, Chen FC, Stoffregen TA. Nintendo Wii balance board is sensitive to effects of visual tasks on standing sway in healthy elderly adults. Gait Posture. 2012;36(3):605–8.

Kurillo G, Chen A, Bajcsy R, Han JJ. Evaluation of upper extremity reachable workspace using Kinect camera. Technol Health Care. 2013;21(6):641–56.

LaViola JJ. Bringing VR and spatial 3D interaction to the masses through video games. IEEE Comput Graph Appl. 2008;28(5):10–5.

Leardini A, Chiari L, Della Croce U, Cappozzo A. Human movement analysis using stereo-photogrammetry. Part 3. Soft tissue artifact assessment and compensation. Gait Posture. 2005;21(2):212–25.

Moore GE. Cramming more components onto integrated circuits. Electronics. 1965;38(8):114–7.

Oh BL, Kim J, Kim J, Hwang JM, Lee J. Validity and reliability of head posture measurement using Microsoft Kinect. Br J Ophthalmol. 2014;98(11):1560–4.

Pagliari D, Pinto L. Calibration of Kinect for Xbox one and comparison between the two generations of Microsoft sensors. Sensors. 2015;15(11):27569–89.

Pfister A, West AM, Bronner S, Noah JA. Comparative abilities of Microsoft Kinect and Vicon 3D motion capture for gait analysis. J Med Eng Technol. 2014;38(5):274–80.

Yeung LF, Cheng KC, Fong CH, Lee WC, Tong KY. Evaluation of the Microsoft Kinect as a clinical assessment tool of body sway. Gait Posture. 2014;40(4):532–8.

Young W, Ferguson S, Brault S, Craig C. Assessing and training standing balance in older adults: a novel approach using the 'Nintendo Wii' balance board. Gait Posture. 2011;33(2):303–5.

Physical Rehabilitation

2

Start by doing what is necessary, then what is possible,
and suddenly you are doing the impossible.

– Saint Francis of Assisi

2.1 Definition and Principles

Before discussing of the use of serious games in rehabilitation, it seems appropriate to define and obtain some precise notions about rehabilitation.

Rehabilitation is a key health strategy to address disability (Meyer et al. 2011).

Rehabilitation is a branch of physical medicine. Rehabilitation, in the area of health, can be defined as the ability to *rehabilitate* patients in his environment: *"the aim of rehabilitation is to restore or return a person to as state of optimal functioning in interaction with his/her environment"* (Meyer et al. 2014). Another interesting definition of the rehabilitation is the one from the World Health Organisation *"a set of measures that assist individuals who experience, or a likely to experience, disability to achieve and maintain optimal functioning in interaction with their environments"* (WHO 2011). Two key elements of the rehabilitation are included in this definition. The first one is the importance of trying to restore optimal functioning of the patient. Of course, unfortunately, in some cases it is not possible to restore "normal" mobility or activity; therefore, rehabilitation is mainly focusing on the function and autonomy during activity of daily living. The second important aspect is the interaction with the environment: interaction with the surrounding objects (move, eat, wash) in order to be as independent as possible but also to interact with people. Social aspect is one of the keys, and unfortunately often neglected, aspect of the rehabilitation and, more generally, of the overall management and integration of disabled people in the society.

© Springer International Publishing AG 2018

B. Bonnechère, *Serious Games in Physical Rehabilitation*,
https://doi.org/10.1007/978-3-319-66122-3_2

2.1.1   A Multidisciplinary Teamwork

Due to the complexity of the pathologies, the rehabilitation is, generally, not performed by a single therapist. Depending on the underlying pathology, a team of specialists are working with the patient to fulfill the best as possible the need and requirement of this particular patient. This expertise from various medical and paramedical points of view is needed in order to have a holistic approach of a particular patient suffering from a specific pathology living in his own environment. It is important to note that two patients presenting the same pathology won't systematically receive the same treatment because lots of parameters have to be taken into consideration (Albert et al. 2012). The International Classification of Functioning, Disability and Health (ICF) from the World Health Organization (WHO) has been created to underline the importance that personal and environmental could and should play in rehabilitation[1].

2.1.1.1 Medical Doctors

The medical doctors involved in the rehabilitation field are, most of the time, doctors in physical medicine and rehabilitation (neurologists can also play the role of team leader). They are responsible of the diagnosis, assess the severity of the disease and the associated troubles and complications. Based on this evaluation, they built a specific rehabilitation program for this specific patient (e.g., Does this patient require occupational therapy? How many sessions of physiotherapy are required? Does this patient need surgery or pharmacological treatment?). During all the rehabilitation process, the doctors control the progress of the patients and, in collaboration with the other professionals in charge of the patient, modify the treatment if needed.

2.1.1.2 Physiotherapists

Physiotherapists are one of the cornerstones of the physical rehabilitation. Generally, it is with physiotherapist that the patients spend most of the rehabilitation time. There are plenty of different techniques, approaches, and philosophies in physiotherapy. Physiotherapists adapt their treatments and exercises depending on the nature of the diseases (neurological, orthopedics). One of the most popular approaches for neurological disease is the neurodevelopment treatment (NDT) (Bobath 1967). The aim of this method is to facilitate the movement by reducing muscle tone and inhibiting primitive and abnormal reflex. Another important aspect of the NDT approach is to allow the patients to have a greater independence and really focus on the movement. We won't list here each technique (details will be provided in Chap. 4). From a scientific point of view, it is important to underline that no particular technique has a higher level of evidence than another one (Kollen et al. 2009). The other important point about physiotherapy and rehabilitation is that the more the patient is moving and performing the exercises the better and faster the progress will be (Langhorne et al. 2011).

---

[1] http://www.who.int/classifications/icf/en/

2.1.1.3 Occupational Therapists

Occupational therapists and physiotherapists are working closely together. Physiotherapists are mainly working on the muscles (e.g., to avoid spasticity) and joints (e.g., to avoid retraction and restoring/preserving enough range of motion); occupational therapists focus their work on (fine) motor function. To summarize roughly, the physiotherapists try to restore enough mobility, and the occupational therapists try to make patients (re)learn some (basic) and functional motion in order to increase their independences (Arbesman et al. 2013). To increase patients' independence, two different, but often complementary, approaches are possible: improving directly the function (in collaboration with physiotherapists) or modifying the environment to allow patient performing these activities, e.g., modify and adopt home environment in order to prevent falls in older people (Pighills et al. 2011), modify the classroom for student with autism (Kinnealey et al. 2012), etc.

2.1.1.4 (Neuro)Psychologists

Depression and anxiety are highly prevalent in patients with chronic diseases, but remain too often undertreated despite significant negative consequences on patient health. Multiple consequences of a chronic disease diagnosis can contribute to depression or anxiety: the loss of a sense of self-worth, anxiety, and uncertainty about the future, loss of relationships and social isolation, and feelings of guilt (Dejean et al. 2013). In the perspective of a more holistic approach of the patient, a psychological and eventually spiritual support must be provided to patient in the early start of the disease (Schulz-Stübner 2007). It is important to note that this psychological support is not only provided by the medical team, the role of the family and relatives is also preponderant (Glass et al. 2004).

2.1.1.5 Speech Therapists

Lesions in the brain (e.g., stroke, cerebral palsy) do not only induce motor problem. Depending on the localization of the primary lesions, some other troubles can be induced. The location of the brain responsible for speech production (Broca's area) and speech comprehension (Wernicke's area) are often affected during stroke. Rehabilitation of the speech, or other communication ways, is thus an important part of the process for some pathology, especially in the light of the definition of the health by the WHO (e.g., optimal interaction with the environment).

2.1.1.6 Prosthetists

The use of prosthesis or medical devices, as temporary or permanent help, aims to give a greater autonomy to patients during activities of daily living and/or rehabilitation session. Depending on the severity of the disability medical devices varied from full support electric wheelchairs in case of severe paraplegia to ankle's brace support to avoid spasticity of the triceps surae during gait in case of light form of spasticity.

For the lower limbs, most orthoses focus on controlling ankle position and kinematic motion during the gait (McNee et al. 2007).

For the upper limbs, the objective is to improve function by increasing the range of motion, limit deformation, and increase functions (Autti-Rämö et al. 2006).

The settings and the optimal functioning of the materials is a team effort including not only the prosthetists but also physiotherapists and occupational therapists. Casting can be an alternative to orthoses in order to increase the efficacy of treatment (e.g., intensive rehabilitation, surgery, botulinum toxin injection) (Hayek et al. 2010).

2.1.1.7 Sports Coach

The definition of the rehabilitation includes *"to achieve and maintain optimal functioning in interaction with their environments"* (WHO 2011). It is therefore obvious that sport should be considered as a complement to the conventional rehabilitation treatment not only for the physical benefits but also for the important and positive effects of the social interaction. Sports for disabled people have been popularized by the huge development and the media coverage of the Paralympic Games. New specialties are emerging in the faculty of physiotherapy or sport sciences in physical activities adapted for people with disabilities.

Important efforts are also done in the development of affordable material (prosthesis, wheelchairs, etc.) to allow disabled people to train and enjoy sport's activities.

Finally, we can also note here the importance that the animals can play during rehabilitation and in particular horses during hippotherapy session.

2.1.1.8 Social Workers

Although only a few people would spontaneously think about social workers in the rehabilitation team, these ones play an important role. Social workers try to solve some obstacles related to rehabilitation (e.g., access to care, financial issues). They also have an important role in the dialogue with the family. They do not only provide material support (access to institution, materials, etc.), they can also be a part on the treatment (e.g., social workers can visit the family to help and support parents with disabled children (Weindling et al. 2007)). This example underlines the fact that the disease affects not only the patient but also his family. It is therefore sometimes interesting to work with family to decrease stress and anxiety level by allowing the patient to evolve in a more favorable environment.

2.1.2 The Neuromusculoskeletal System

The general aim of rehabilitation is to restore or return a person to a state of optimal functioning. For achieving this goal, different objectives are targeted such as posture, balance, strength, coordination, endurance, and dexterity.

For a healthy subject, a lot of daily activities are done automatically, without even thinking about it, despite this "automation" even a relatively simple motion such as taking a glass and drinking it required optimal functioning and the synchronization of a lot of systems. It is interesting to have an overview of this complex system in order to understand the pathologies, and therefore the different strategies of rehabilitation. Here is a (non-exhaustive and simplified) list of the principle component of the nervous and musculoskeletal system involved in voluntary contraction.

We try to schematize all these information in Fig. 2.1 with the main function of each component and few examples of pathologies that can affect each level.

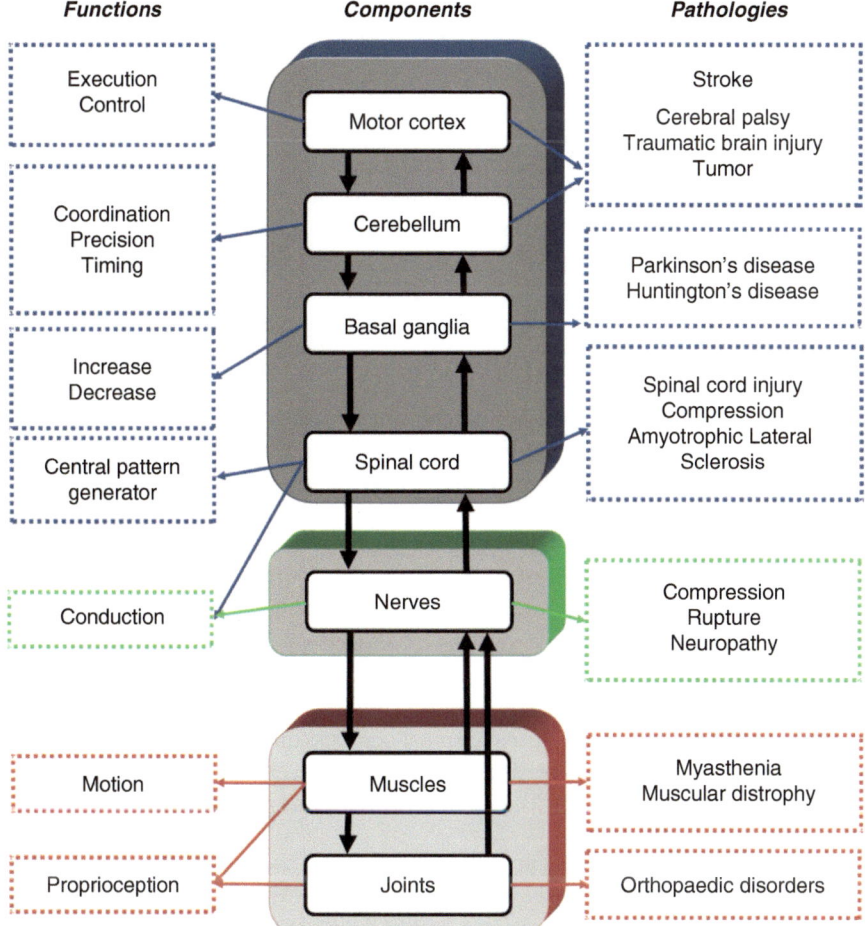

Fig. 2.1 From brain to muscles: a simplified view of the different component involved in voluntary contraction. *Blue color* is for central nervous system, *green color* is for the peripheral nervous system, and *red color* is for the musculoskeletal system. *Left column* summarized main functions of each component, *right* one lists major pathologies concerning each levels

- Central nervous system (CNS)
  - The motor cortex: Located in the frontal lobe, it is involved in the programming (mainly in the premotor cortex that is located in front of the motor cortex), the execution and the control of voluntary movement. Lesions (e.g., stroke, traumatic brain injury, tumors) in the motor cortex induce paralysis. The motor cortex is composed by different components: the primary motor cortex, the premotor cortex, the supplementary motor cortex, and the posterior parietal cortex.
  - The cerebellum: Involved in the coordination, precision, and accurate timing of the motion. The cerebellum is important in the acquisition and learning of new skills and motricity. It allows supervised learning of a new task by transmitting the error between the expected motion and the performed one to the motor cortex: it's a feedforward learning. Therefore, a lesion in the cerebellum induces posture and balance disorders, difficulties with motor learning and fine movement controls (dexterity). The cerebellum has also an important cognitive function mainly for the language and the attention.
  - The basal ganglia: Acts like an inhibitor for motor systems, when this inhibition is released the motor system is activated. The basal ganglia also play a role in the acquisition of new skills: it's involved in the reinforcement learning. Lesions in the basal ganglia induce trouble in motor control, mainly hyperkinetic disorders (e.g., difficulty to initiate movement in Parkinson's disease, difficulty to prevent unintentional movement in Huntington's disease).
  - The spinal cord: Makes the link between the CNS and the peripheral nerves. Relays information from brain to muscles through the efferent or descending pathways (pyramidal and extrapyramidal tracts) and from peripheral (muscles, joints, glands, organs) to brain through the afferent or ascending pathways (dorsal column medial lemniscus system, spinocerebellar tracts, anterolateral system). Patients with spinal cord injuries could present various symptomatologies depending on the severity and localization of the lesions: from muscle weakness and loss of sensitivity within limited regions (i.e., herniated disc) to full body paralysis (i.e., laceration of the spinal cord in the cervical spine due to trauma).
- Peripheral nervous system
  - The nerves: Relays between the spinal cord and the muscles, joints, ligaments, bones, etc. Nerves can be stretched, compressed, cut inducing muscles' weakness or paralysis (efferent), loss of sensitivity, and proprioception (afferent).
- Musculoskeletal system
  - The muscles: Muscles' contraction is a complex mechanism involving neuromuscular junction (release of neurotransmitter [mainly acetylcholine]) and the slide of myo-filaments (actin and myosin) to produce changes in muscles' lengths and finally producing motion. The muscle spindles also provide information to the CNS relative to the length and the stretch of the muscle; those information are called proprioception. In rehabilitation, it is important to restore or preserve the proprioception to maintain optimal functioning of the musculoskeletal system (fine motor function and balance). The muscles are attached to bones by tendons (also containing proprioceptive fibers).

– The joints: Movement can be defined as the change of position of one bone related to another one. Bones are linked together through joints; these joints are reinforced by ligaments. Ligaments provide lots of proprioceptive information (avoiding luxation of the joint).

2.1.3   Treatment and Exercises

Depending on the level of the lesions (cerebellum, spinal cord) and the severity of the disease (e.g., moderate balance problem due to lack of vascularization of the cerebellum, quadriplegia in case of complete spinal cord injury), the objectives and techniques of rehabilitation are totally different.

General aim of the rehabilitation is to increase muscle coordination; reduce muscle weakness and/or muscle tone; improve balance; improve gait and motion independence; limit bone deformation and bone deviation.

There is one constant in every rehabilitation program: the more the patient is performing the exercises the more efficient the program will be (Langhorne et al. 2011). Therefore, the rehabilitation does not only take place during the supervised sessions with the clinicians, patients also need to perform some exercises alone (at home, in the room, etc.). To be efficient these exercises must be performed and most important there must be well achieved. If the exercises are not well performed (inability to perform alone due to the disability, patient forget how to perform correctly the exercises), it can lead to some perverse adverse effects: increase of compensatory movements, vicious posture, etc.

Therefore, it is important to have a regular feedback between clinicians and patients to ensure that the patients are performing the exercises and that they are doing them correctly.

Depending on the pathology, the age of the patient, the infrastructure, etc., the number and durations of the session varies between several sessions a day (in specialized center in case of severe disability) to one weekly session.

2.2   Obstacles to Rehabilitation

The road to a successful rehabilitation is long and difficult. A lot of obstacles can interfere with this rehabilitation. It is important to be aware of those problems in order to try to develop and find efficient solutions. A systematic review on the treatment adherence identified four groups of barriers; the following points are strongly associated with a lower adherence to treatment (Jack et al. 2010) and therefore a lower success of the rehabilitation:

• Physical
    – Low level of physical activity at aerobic capacity at baseline
    – Low in-treatment adherence with exercise
    – Low level of exercise adherence in previous weeks

- Psychological
  - Low self-efficacy (for exercises, task, and coping)
  - High level of depression at the beginning of the treatment (baseline)
  - No change or worse depression compared with baseline
  - High degree of helplessness
- Sociodemographic
  - Poor social or family support for activity
  - Greater number of barriers to exercise
- Clinical
  - Worsening of pain during exercise

Note that most of the studies included in this review were about orthopedic disorders (osteoarthritis, low back pain). Instead of these four categories, we identify five different groups of obstacle:

2.2.1   Severity of the Disease

It is not only the severity of the disease that matters but mainly the possibility of evolution that is overriding the rehabilitation process. Concerning neurological diseases, most pathologies are non-curative: when neurological cells are damaged, most of the time by defect of vascularization (stroke), there is currently no possibility of repairing or implanting new cells (research works on stem cells are not advanced enough yet). Despite the huge number of cells that constitute the brain, approximately 10 billion of neurons supported by 100 billion glial cells, brain plasticity (i.e., establishing new connections between neurons) is very complex and those mechanisms are still poorly understood in fundamental research (Small et al. 2013) and therefore not ready to be implemented in clinics yet.

Concerning the peripheral nerves, the regeneration is depending on the type of the nerves (with or without myelin sheath). In the best cases, nerves can grow about 1 mm a day (Mowery et al. 2014).

Other pathologies such as Parkinson's disease, lateral amyotrophic sclerosis, or multiple sclerosis are progressive diseases: the state of the patients is slowly decreasing.

Rehabilitation must then focus on improving the capacity of the patient with nonprogressive disease, trying to find alternative way of moving, etc. Keeping in mind that previous condition will never be reached again, patients must of course be informed of the objectives of the different phases of treatment to understand the goals and improve the adherence to treatment (see Chap. 3).

In case of progressive diseases, rehabilitation focuses on avoiding the effects of the disease to decrease the underlying disability and increase patient's autonomy.

2.2.2 Motivational Issues

Patient's motivation is obviously an important factor to take into consideration since patients, and more particularly young patients (e.g., children suffering from cerebral palsy), must perform as many rehabilitation exercises as possible.

> *"Lack of motivation is one of the most frequently cited reasons for patient dropout, failure to comply, relapse, and other negative treatment outcomes."* (Ryan and Plant 1995).

For some pathologies (see Chap. 4), rehabilitation schemes are advised on a frequent basis.

Therefore the motivation of the patients is the main key to as successful rehabilitation treatment (Deutsch et al. 2008). The main challenge is therefore to keep patients motivated enough despite the feeling he/she could have of "inefficiency," "lack of progress," "tiredness," etc. Such problems are even more present with teenagers during the puberty identity crisis. Even if progresses are very slow, or that the patient feels that there is no progress at all, it is important for him to continue rehabilitation program. If not his condition could deteriorate and the patient can lose the benefits of the previous sessions. This quote of Mahatma Gandhi perfectly represents this situation:

> *"Whatever you do will be insignificant, but it is very important that you do it."*

2.2.3 Financial Issues

Ideally, financial issues should not be an obstacle for the management of health-related problems. This is unfortunately not the case and depending on the national health system of the country (if any!) the part of the treatment that the patient must pay could definitely be an obstacle for some patients. Due to the non-standardization of national health system and costs associated to treatment in different countries, it is impossible to quantify the price paid by the patient. Table 2.1 quantifies the interventions defined hereabove without intervention of national health care system. A huge gap exists between North and South countries (developed and emerging countries) concerning poverty. Poverty is not just a financial state; it affects health, education, life expectancy, and quality of life. The problems related to access to care are important and should not be neglected when developing new solutions for rehabilitation in order to not further increase the gap between the different countries.

2.2.4 Access to Care

There are two kinds of potential issues related to access to care (apart from the financial problems already mentioned).

Table 2.1 Prices of various medical and paramedical interventions (in Belgium without intervention of the national health system).

	Euro	US dollar
Medical doctor		
General practitioner	25€	35$
Specialist	45€	62$
Physiotherapy		
Per session (depending on the duration)	22–70€	30–100$
Evaluation	60–300€	80–400$
Occupational therapy		
Per session	20€	28$
Observational evaluation	150€	207$
Psychology		
Per session	20–50€	28–70$
Speech therapy		
Per session	22€	30$
Prosthesis and medical device		
Manual wheelchair	700–2000€	965–2760$
Electric wheelchair	5000–10,000€	7000–14,000$
Ankle orthoses	50–150€	70–207$
Knee orthoses	150–500€	207–690$
Wrist orthoses	70–150€	100–207$
Shoulder orthoses	100–500€	138–690$

The first one is that the patients need to be close to a rehabilitation center or clinicians. Lack of access to available rehabilitation services, especially in low-income countries or rural areas, has been pinpointed as a major barrier to rehabilitation by the WHO (WHO 2011). The density of physicians working in different regions of the world is highly inhomogeneous. The Caribbean Island of Cuba has more number of physicians per person working there; less number of physicians per person are in the Southeastern African territory of Malawi. In 2004, there were 7.7 million physicians working around the world. A large number of physicians were in China, which is the largest territory on the map. If physicians were distributed according to population, there would be 124 physicians to every 100,000 people. The most concentrated 50% of physicians live in territories with less than one fifth of the world's population. The worst off fifth are served by only 2% of the world's physicians.[2]

For intervention that does not require rehabilitation material clinicians can visit patients in their home.

Access to specific medical device (MRI, Pet-Scan) is limited to specialized center that may be inaccessible to patients (distance, no public transport available, no transport adapted for disabled people).

---

[2] www.worldmapper.org

The second one is really about the "physical" accessibility to clinicians and/or rehabilitation center. New constructions are built following norms and are therefore, supposed to be, adapted (doors, elevator, height of the switch, toilet) for disabled people (especially in clinical center).

The problem of access to care is not only limited to the access of the clinical center but it includes all the journey between patient's home and this center; existence of sidewalk adapted for wheelchairs, access for people with crutches, with walkers, public transport adapted and accessible, inclined plane instead of stairs. In this domain, lots of efforts still need to be taken.

2.2.5   Lack of Time

Situation is different for each patient (children, workers, unemployed). However, it is known that approximately only 30% of the patients, suffering mainly of orthopedics disease, are performing rehabilitation exercises at home as recommended by their physiotherapists.

To our best knowledge, such kind of data are not available for patients suffering from neurological diseases for whom performing exercises at home is at least important for orthopedics patients.

The second reason cited for not performing the exercises at home is lack of time. If patients are not taking 15 min per day to perform exercises at home, they will have the difficulty to find at least 1 h (one rehabilitation session is approximately 30 min plus the transport) for going to the rehabilitation center.

2.3   Telemedicine and E-Health

Thanks to the development of the technology (see Chap. 1), in particular the Internet, a new branch of medicine has emerged: the telemedicine.

Although telemedicine is closely associated to technology, it is interesting to note that the first telemedicine consultations were performed in 1920! It was literally a medical consultation on the phone. However, we cannot really consider this as telemedicine, in its current form at least.

WHO defines telemedicine as *"The delivery of health care service, where distance is a critical factor, by all care professionals using information and telecommunication technologies for the exchange of valid information for diagnosis, treatment and prevention of disease and injury, research and evaluation, and for the continuing education of health care providers, all in the interests of advancing the health of individuals and their communities."* (WHO 1998)

There are three different sides in telemedicine: the first two are commonly used in daily clinical practice[3].

---

[3] http://www.americantelemed.org/learn/what-is-telemedicine

- The interactive telemedicine provides real-time interaction between patients and clinicians by phone calls, video conference, etc. Clinical history and psychological examination can be easily conducted with interactive telemedicine (Currell et al. 2000).
- The store and forward telemedicine: the medical data such as radiography, electrocardiography, and motion analysis are recorded, stored, and then analyzed later on by a doctor.
- The remote patient monitoring is the device used to remotely collect data at patient's home. These data are then sent, stored, and analyzed to control patients. Depending on the pathology, a large number of variables can be controlled such as heart rates, blood pressure, blood glucose, and weight. When these variables present abnormalities, the patient is contacted by a nurse or the doctor and a consultation can be planned.

Telemedicine could be an alternative to face-to-face approaches to reduce costs, increase geographic accessibility, or act as a mechanism to extend limited resources (McCue et al. 2010).

One of the branches of the telemedicine is telerehabilitation. *"The Telerehabilitation refers to the delivery of rehabilitation services via information and communication technologies. Clinically, this term encompasses a range of rehabilitation and habilitation services that include assessment, monitoring, prevention, intervention, supervision, education, consultation, and counseling. Telerehabilitation services are delivered to adults and children by a broad range of professionals that may include, but is not limited to, physical therapists, speech-language pathologists, occupational therapists, audiologists, rehabilitation physicians and nurses, rehabilitation engineers, assistive technologists, teachers, psychologists, and dieticians. As other personnel such as paraprofessionals, family members, and caregivers may assist during telerehabilitation sessions"*[4]

Telerehabilitation is a new field and thus it is difficult, currently, to evaluate the possibilities and limits of this new approach. In a recent review, 19 studies on rehabilitation for any disability associated with a neurological deficit or condition were evaluated. In 13 studies, the telerehabilitation was successful in providing at least equivalent outcomes to conventional approach (Hailey et al. 2013).

Chapter 4 will focus on the serious games, one discipline of the telemedicine and telerehabilitation.

---

[4]A Blueprint for Telerehabilitation Guidelines, The American Telemedicine Association, 2010

References

Albert T, Beuret Blanquart F, Le Chapelain L, Fattal C, Goossens D, Rome J, Yelnik AP, Perrouin Verbe B, French Physical and Rehabilitation Medicine Society, French Federation of PRM. Physical and rehabilitation medicine (PRM) care pathways: "spinal cord injury". Ann Phys Rehabil Med. 2012;55(6):440–50.

Arbesman M, Bazyk S, Nochajski SM. Systematic review of occupational therapy and mental health promotion, prevention, and intervention for children and youth. Am J Occup Ther. 2013;67(6):e120–30.

Autti-Rämö I, Suoranta J, Anttila H, Malmivaara A, Mäkelä M. Effectiveness of upper and lower limb casting and orthoses in children with cerebral palsy: an overview of review articles. Am J Phys Med Rehabil. 2006;85(1):89–103.

Bobath B. The very early treatment of cerebral palsy. Dev Med Child Neurol. 1967;9:373–90.

Currell R, Urquhart C, Wainwright P, Lewis R. Telemedicine versus face to face patient care: effects on professional practice and health care outcomes. Cochrane Database Syst Rev. 2000;2:CD002098.

Dejean D, Giacomini M, Vanstone M, Brundisini F. Patient experiences of depression and anxiety with chronic disease: a systematic review and qualitative meta-synthesis. Ont Health Technol Assess Ser. 2013;13(16):1–33.

Deutsch JE, Borbely M, Filler J, Guarrera-Bowlby KH. Use of a low-cost, commercially available gaming console (Wii) for rehabilitation of an adolescent with cerebral palsy. Phys Ther. 2008;88(10):1196–207.

Glass TA, Berkman LF, Hiltunen EF, Furie K, Glymour MM, Fay ME, Ware J. The families in recovery from stroke trial (FIRST): primary study results. Psychosom Med. 2004;66(6):889–97.

Hailey D, Roine R, Ohinmaa A, Dennett L. The status of telerehabilitation in neurological applications. J Telemed Telecare. 2013;19(6):307–10.

Hayek S, Gershon A, Wientroub S, Yizhar Z. The effect of injections of botulinum toxin type a combined with casting on the equinus gait of children with cerebral palsy. J Bone Joint Surg Br. 2010;92(8):1152–9.

Jack K, McLean SM, Moffett JK, Gardiner E. Barriers to treatment adherence in physiotherapy outpatient clinics: a systematic review. Man Ther. 2010;15(3):220–8.

Kinnealey M, Pfeiffer B, Miller J, Roan C, Shoener R, Ellner ML. Effect of classroom modification on attention and engagement of students with autism or dyspraxia. Am J Occup Ther. 2012;66(5):511–9.

Kollen BJ, Lennon S, Lyons B, Wheatley-Smith L, Scheper M, Buurke JH, Halfens J, Geurts AC, Kwakkel G. The effectiveness of the Bobath concept in stroke rehabilitation: what is the evidence? Stroke. 2009;40(4):e89–97.

Langhorne P, Bernhardt J, Kwakkel G. Stroke rehabilitation. Lancet. 2011;377(9778):1693–702.

McCue M, Fairman A, Pramuka M. Enhancing quality of life through telerehabilitation. Phys Med Rehabil Clin N Am. 2010;21(1):195–205.

McNee AE, Will E, Liu JP, Eve LC, Gough M, Morrissey MC, Shortland AP. The effect of serial casting on gait in children with cerebral palsy: preliminary results from a crossover trial. Gait Posture. 2007;25(3):463–8.

Meyer T, Gutenbrunner C, Bickenbach J, Cieza A, Melvin J, Stucki G. Towards a shared conceptual description of rehabilitation as a health strategy. J Rehabil Med. 2011;43:765–9.

Meyer T, Gutenbrunner C, Kiekens C, Skempes D, Melvin JL, Schedler K, Imamura M, Stucki G. ISPRM discussion paper: proposing a conceptual description of health-related rehabilitation services. J Rehabil Med. 2014;46(1):1–6.

Mowery TM, Kostylev PV, Garraghty PE. AMPA and GABAA/B receptor subunit expression in the cuneate nucleus of adult squirrel monkeys during peripheral nerve regeneration. Neurosci Lett. 2014;559:141–6.

Pighills AC, Torgerson DJ, Sheldon TA, Drummond AE, Bland JM. Environmental assessment and modification to prevent falls in older people. J Am Geriatr Soc. 2011;59(1):26–33.

Ryan RM, Plant RW. Initial motivations for alcohol treatment: relations with patient characteristics, treatment involvement, and dropout. Science. 1995;20(3):279–97.

Schulz-Stübner S. Intensive care unit management of patients with stroke. Curr Treat Options Neurol. 2007;9(6):427–41.

Small SL, Buccino G, Solodkin A. Brain repair after stroke-a novel neurological model. Nat Rev Neurol. 2013;9(12):698–707.

Weindling AM, Cunningham CC, Glenn SM, Edwards RT, Reeves DJ. Additional therapy for young children with spastic cerebral palsy: a randomised controlled trial. Health Technol Assess. 2007;11(16):iii–v; ix-x, 1–71

World Health Organization (WHO). A health telematics policy in support of WHO's health-for-all strategy for global health development: report of the WHO group consultation on health telematics. Geneva: WHO; 1998.

World Health Organization (WHO). World Health Organization (WHO) & World Bank world report on disability. Geneva: WHO; 2011.

The (Serious) Games

3

When you strip away the genre differences and the technological
complexities, all games share four defining traits: a goal, rules,
a feedback system, and voluntary participation.

– McGonigal Jane

3.1 The Games in the Society

Since the dawn of time, games have always been present and play an important role in the society for the development of the children, for social and psychomotor development, for teaching purpose, for adults, social cohesion, learning, etc. Since 1950, a distinction has been done between the "traditional games" and video games.

3.1.1 Traditional Games

The first traces of board gaming equipments were found in Iraq and are back to 3000 BC. This game was called the Royal Game of Ur. Games were also found in Egypt (*Senet*), China (*Wei-qui*), and in Japan (*Go*) between 3000 and 2000 BC.

Some games, still played today, have a long history. Around Jesus Christ some records of the Emperor Claudius playing Tabula, an early version of Backgammon were found. Chess game was created in India around the years 600 AD. Card games are mentioned in Europe for the first time during the year 1300 AD, and the first standard cart suits (heart, clubs, spades, and diamonds) was created in France in 1480. Bridge and Poker were then both developed during the 1800s. The development of one of the most popular games: the Monopoly is representative of the combined aspects of the games: having fun and learning something at the same time. This game has indeed been developed to illustrate the negative effect of concentrating land in private monopolies (the single tax theory) (Orbanes 2006). This game,

© Springer International Publishing AG 2018
B. Bonnechère, *Serious Games in Physical Rehabilitation*,
https://doi.org/10.1007/978-3-319-66122-3_3

called the Landlord's game, was developed in 1903 and has been commercialized by Parker Brothers as Monopoly from 1935. Another popular game: the Scrabble was invented in 1931 (*Lexico*) and commercialized as Scrabble in 1947.

There are several different kinds of games: some can be played alone (*patience card games*), some are based on strategy (*Stratego*) and skills (*Risk*) while others are only based on chance (*Blackjack*).

Games can also be classified according to the purpose: memory (*Concentration or Pairs card games*), speed and dexterity (*Jenga*), coordination (a*ir hockey*).

3.1.2   Video Games

> Computer games don't affect kids; I mean if Pac-Man affected us as kids, we'd all been running around in darkened rooms, munching magic pills and listening to repetitive electronic music.
>
> – Wilson Kristian, CEO of Nintendo

It is estimated that 97% of children and adolescents in the United States of America play video games at least 1 h per day (Granic et al. 2014). In 2009, the average was 1 h and 13 min every day, a nearly threefold increase from 10 years earlier[1]!

Video, or computer, games have more detractors than partisans! Those in favor of video games highlighted the fact that games improve dexterity, management, and could be beneficial for the brain. While people against computer games emphasize the fact that games promote violence, obesity, and decrease in social life. In this chapter, we are going to analyze what is the current level of evidence of each of those points.

3.1.2.1 Pro's

Depending on the kind of games played (simulation, strategy, role-playing, war), several skills could be trained with video games.

Dexterity

Regular practice of video games, especially when the player is immersed in a three-dimensional environment, could have positive impact on the dexterity of surgeons. This is particularly true for the laparoscopic surgery (surgical technique using a laparoscope [optic cable system] to view the affected area and haptic grippers to perform the surgery). In this case, the 3D real environment (body of the patient) is projected on a screen in 2D, video games help the surgeons to evaluate distances and perspectives in this particular environment. It is interesting to note that the correlation between the video game performance and laparoscopic skills was significant and positive, but not between video game performance and traditional surgical skills scores (Millard et al. 2014). Based on those studies, laparoscopic simulators have been developed to prepare surgeons before their surgeries (Willis et al. 2014).

---

[1] http://kaiserfamilyfoundation.files.wordpress.com/2013/01/8010.pdf.

Some researchers have also highlighted that performing some warm-up with serious games before the surgery was beneficial for the patients (Jalink et al. 2015).

It has also been demonstrated that playing action video games could increase oculomotor performance of the players (West et al. 2013).

Management

Many games are based on strategy and management. Here are some examples of role-playing and strategy games; players must build and manage a city in SimCity, an airport in Airport Simulator, a farm in Farmy Simulator, etc. Therefore, some researchers have proposed that video games could develop good learning principles and may promote problem-solving skills. A positive correlation has been found between strategic video game play and the self-reported problem-solving skills with adolescents (Adachi and Willoughby 2013). These authors concluded that strategic video games promote self-reported problem-solving skills and indirectly predict academic grades. Those points are important considering that millions of adolescents play video games every day.

Mental Training

Mental training is an exercise of the mind in order to reach a desired physical result[2]. This approach is used by a lot of sportsman to prepare a race or train a particular movement (e.g., the skiers who is mimicking the course before starting, eyes closed, with his arms). There are different techniques in the mental training: the goal setting, the positive self-talk, and the imagery (Arvinen-Barrow et al. 2015). A regular training with simulator games, sports game but also flight or train simulator, is beneficial for goal setting and mental imagery. Those simulators are used by the students to practice before the real-world situation. Since a few years, race car simulators have been even used to detect new talents. The winner of the virtual competition receives indeed a professional training and is competing in the real championship the following year. This is the best example of how to transfer virtual ability to reality[3].

Playing video games could also have a positive effect on speed reaction time. Action video games (i.e., first person shooter games) require the players to develop the ability to quickly analyze situation, monitor fast moving (enemies) and inhibit erroneous action (don't shoot on your allies). Current research seems to support that action video games are associated with enhanced flexible updating of task-relevant information without affecting impulsivity of the players (Colzato et al. 2013).

Cognition

Playing video games could also be beneficial for the brain and the cognitive function in particular with elderly subjects: games appear to offset declines in age-sensitive cognitive function (Whitbourne et al. 2013). As any kind of repeated

---

[2] http://www.uniquemindesp.info/index.php?option=com_content&view=article&id=772&Itemid=1150.

[3] http://www.nissanusa.com/gtacademyshow/.

activity (e.g., sport training, rehabilitation), regular video games playing/training induce brain spasticity in adolescents (Kühn et al. 2011) but also in adults (Kühn and Gallinat 2014). There is a positive correlation between the amount of video gaming and the increase of gray matter volume of the brain.

It is important to mention here that all games do not have positive effect on the cognitive function. There is, currently, no consensus in the scientific community to determine the best kind of video games to develop cognitive function.

For some authors, the entorhinal cortex volume (part of the brain involved in memory and olfaction) can be predicted by the kind of video game played. Logic/ puzzle games and platform games seem to contribute positively and action-based role-playing games contribute negatively (Kühn et al. 2011). On the other hand a meta-analysis concluded that shooter video game improved spatial skills and these improvements were similar to the effects of lectures (high school or university level). A very interesting point is that the authors also concluded that the skills acquired during the games can be transferred to activity of daily living (Granic et al. 2014).

The famous games "Dr Kawashima's Brain Training: How Old Is Your Brain®" could therefore really be positive for the brain, but not only this kind of games. Actually, it seems that playing shooter games is even more efficient to enhance cognitive function than puzzle or role-playing game (Green and Bavelier 2012).

Social Life

This point will also be discussed more in detail in the Chap. 4 because it is mainly considered as a negative outcome of the games.

However some people, surprisingly, mainly elderly and aged players, explained that playing video games is a good way to stay socially active (Whitbourne et al. 2013). There have been major modifications in the last 20 years in the way of playing video games, and currently the average gamer is not socially isolated. Approximately, 70% of the gamers play with friends online or directly together.[4]

The different kinds of social interactions related to the type of games are presented in Fig. 3.1.

Phobia

Patients suffering from phobia (arachnophobia, fear of flying, aerophobia, claustrophobia, etc.) can be helped by video games (Malbos et al. 2008; Rus-Calafell et al. 2013). The games slowly recreate the patient's fear in the virtual environment step by step.

Another important health-related issue that could be potentially treated by video games is the Post-Traumatic Stress Disorder (PTSD). Lots of studies have been done with war veterans; virtual reality treatment is associated with a reduction of PTSD (Rothbaum et al. 2014).

Games could also be used by patient with autism spectrum disorders in order to reduce fear, anxiety level, and to increase social skills (Maskey et al. 2014).

---

[4] http://www.theesa.ca/wp-content/uploads/2012/10/ESAC_ESSENTIAL_FACTS_2012_EN.pdf.

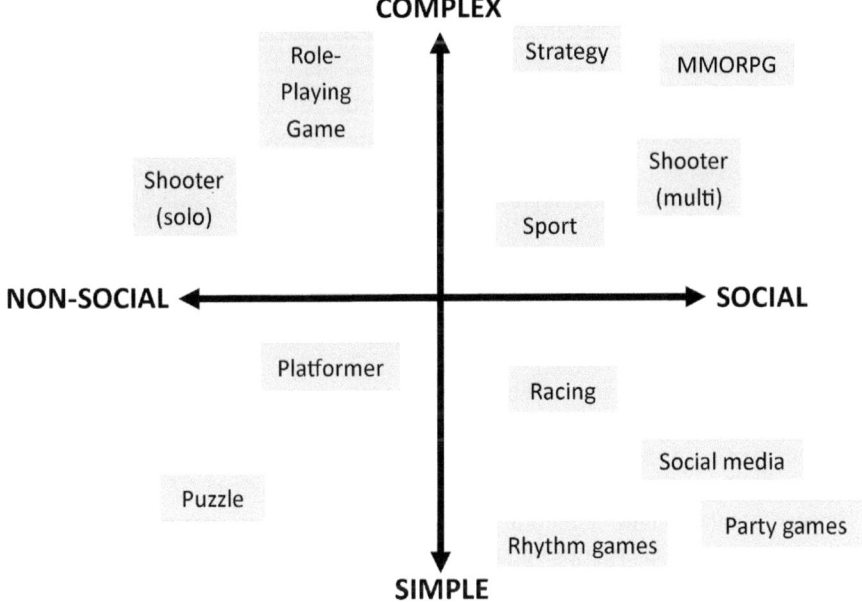

Fig. 3.1 The different kinds of video games and their relations with social interaction (adapted from Granic et al. 2014). *MMORPG* Massively Multiplayer Online Role Playing Games

Virtual reality could also be used as a diagnostic tool for PTSD patients; it seems indeed that players' physiological measurements (heart rate, respiratory rate, skin conductance, etc.) and reaction during games could be used to detect people with higher risk of suffering from PTS (Costanzo et al. 2014).

3.1.2.2 Contra's

Violence and Aggressiveness

The U.S. Supreme Court ruled that video games enjoy full free speech protections and that the regulation of violent game sales to minors is unconstitutional. The Supreme Court also referred to psychological research on violent video games as "unpersuasive" and noted that such research contains many methodological flaws. Recent reviews in many scholarly journals have come to similar conclusions although much debate continues (Ferguson 2013).

This is indeed an old debate and, despite the fact that the U.S. Supreme Court held that the studies linking violence and video games presented methodological flaws, there are much more studies highlighting an increase of violence due to frequent use of violent video games than the opposite.

Actually the problem of violence is broader and should not be limited to video games only but also include movies, video-media-televisions, music clips, games, the Internet, and social media become the primary model for transmitting aggressiveness to children (Cardwell 2013).

Different theories have been developed to explain the link between violent video games and the level of aggressiveness of the players. One of the most popular theories is that violent video games are stressful (e.g., explosions, enemies trying to kill you) and it has been demonstrated that the stress increases the aggressivity. A group of researchers has compared the level of stress and aggressiveness when playing violent and nonviolent games. As expected, violent video game players had higher stress level and aggression level than nonviolent game players (Hasan et al. 2013).

Yet, as mentioned above, authors did not all agree on this relationship. After testing several kinds of games (violent, nonviolent, or prosocial), researchers failed to prove that playing any kind of video games affects prosocial behavior (Tear and Nielsen 2013).

Another popular theory is that some players, people with pre-existing mental health problem, could be affected more by the violent games. A population of 377 children presenting attention deficit or depressive symptoms was included in a study to test this hypothesis. Results did not support the hypothesis that children with elevated mental health symptoms constitute a "vulnerable" population for video game violence effects (Ferguson and Olson 2014).

In conclusion, it seems not possible to have a final stance on the issue but it is important to be aware that increased aggressivity can be linked to several sources of media, not only video games, and affects various people with different conditions in a variety of ways (Hoffman 2014).

Obesity, Overweight, and Decreased Physical Activity Level
Due to the evolution of games controllers, a distinction needs to be done between active and sedentary (passive) video games. First, we are going to discuss the sedentary video games because there are still, currently, the more popular and used compared to active ones.

It is obvious that watching television and playing video games seated in a sofa—eventually drinking soda and eating chips—is an, almost perfect, example of sedentary behavior that increases the risk of overweight, hypertension, and diabetes. The total screen time for adolescents (11–17 years old) is 4.5 ± 2.4 h/day (Baer et al. 2012). Once again a distinction must be done between the different kinds of games played. A study has been done to compare three different conditions: violent video games, competitive nonviolent game, or watching TV. The studied variables were: blood pressure, appetite perception, and food preferences. Violent video game playing was associated with a significant increase in diastolic blood pressure compared with the other two groups. Subjects playing violent video games felt less full and reported a tendency towards sweet food consumption. Video games involving violence appear to be associated with significant effects on blood pressure, food preference, and appetite perceptions compared with nonviolent gaming or watching TV (Siervo et al. 2013).

As expected, there is a positive association between the Body Mass Index (BMI) and the time spent on the Internet or video games by boys. There is also a greater proportion of obese boys spending more than 2 h daily in front of the screen. The time spent playing outside after school is negatively associated with BMI. Note that these observations are not true for girls (Gates et al. 2013).

The same relation is found with adults; it is striking to note that playing only more than once a week is sufficient to increase the risk of being overweight. Contrariwise, no significant association was found between the Internet use and overweight (Melchior et al. 2014).

In addition to the overweight problem, spending too much time in front of a screen (Internet, TV, video games) is associated with a lot of other troubles such as bullying, being bullied, decreased physical activity level, skipping school, alcohol use, and unhealthy eating habits. Compulsive and excessive screen times are associated with several psychosocial problems (Busch et al. 2013).

Most children and youth around the world do not meet current physical activity guidelines and are considered to be inactive by WHO (2010). According to those guidelines, the minimum daily physical activity duration is 60 min of moderate-to-vigorous intensity activities (Spinks et al. 2007).

In order to fight against the sedentary lifestyle of young people and especially frequent video players, video games companies have introduced new games controllers to turn the players more active (e.g., The Nintendo Wii™ and the Microsoft Xbox Kinect™).

Is it working and is it enough to fight against sedentary lifestyle? Playing active video games induce indeed a significant increase of energy expenditure compared to a rest situation (i.e., sitting in the sofa playing sedentary games). But the level of energy expenditure is rather low and there is no significant difference between playing video games and walking. The amount of energy expenditure is depending on the games but, unfortunately, active video games are not intense enough to contribute towards the 60 min daily moderate-to-vigorous physical activity that is recommended for children by WHO (White et al. 2011).

Unfortunately, the ratio between active and passive video games is still in favor of the passive one. It is estimated that 24% of adults and 41% of children are playing active video games. Adults spend playing 33% of their time in active video games and nearly 20% of children in video games(Fullerton et al. 2014).

Note that the use of commercial and serious games to fight against overweight and obesity is discussed in Sect. 4.3.

One last point that needs to be addressed is whether or not the use of these games is associated with an increase of energy intake in which case the benefit associated with these games would be null or even negative! This is not the case and there is no difference in terms of "snacking" between active and sedentary games. However, it should be noted that the energy intake while playing video games, active or passive, is 166% more than the calories required during resting conditions (Mellecker et al. 2010). Therefore, the balance between energy intake and expenditure while playing video games is not in favor of the players.

Social Life

We have seen that 97% of children and adolescents in the States play video games at least 1 h per day (Granic et al. 2014). When the players were asked what sacrifices they are ready to make to play computer games; 25% responded "another hobby," 20% "socializing with friends, family and/or partner" or "sleep" and less than 10% said "work and/or education" (Griffiths et al. 2004).

Currently, majority of the games are being played online in cooperative or competitive mode. The Massive Multiplayer Online Role-Playing Games (MMORPG) are becoming more and more popular and this kind of games require social cooperation and communication, at least virtually; this could be a positive point. But it is interesting to note that this social support, through the Internet, is done at the expense of real physical contacts. Indeed, video game players reported that they received less social support from family members and friends and that they perceived the Internet community as a positive social support (Weaver et al. 2009).

Another potential negative effect is the fact that playing video games induces sleep perturbation and affects negatively the quality of sleep (Exelmans and Van den Bulck 2015).

Acute Injury
Turning the player into a more active person is beneficial for the energy expenditure but it could have adverse effects. Like regular sport training, an intensive "training" in active video games can induce some injuries. Several accidents, mainly case-reports, have been published in the literature. Most of the complaints concern minor musculoskeletal disorders (e.g., tendinitis). On the other side, several accidents have been reported such as a patient who presented an acute strangulation of a pre-existing asymptomatic paraumbilical hernia after completing a series of aerobic exercises on the Wii Fit (Khan et al. 2013), the case of a self-inflicted penetrating eye injury, late retinal detachment, and vision loss in a 7-year-old boy resulting from the use of a Wii Remote (Razavi and Lam 2011), a case of arm swelling with associated rise in serum creatine kinase to over 8000 U/L in a man, following unaccustomed and sustained strenuous muscle exertion through the use of the Nintendo Wii (Baxter and Madhok 2011), a case of forehead laceration (Wells 2008), a case of a severe thumb bone injury (Galanopoulos et al. 2012), a patellar dislocation (Hirpara and Abouazza 2008), a traumatic hemothorax (Peek et al. 2008), and an acute tendinitis of shoulder muscle (Bonis 2007).

3.2   Games in Rehabilitation

The use of traditional games in rehabilitation has been investigated for decades by psychologists and physiotherapists.

Several theories have been developed to explain social and cognitive development through games and play (e.g., Piaget 1962; Gottman 1986). Piaget's theory explained that make-believe play provides players the opportunity to reproduce real-life conflict and ameliorate negative feeling.

Gottman emphasized that play constitutes an emotionally significant context through which pain loss and anxiety can be enacted.

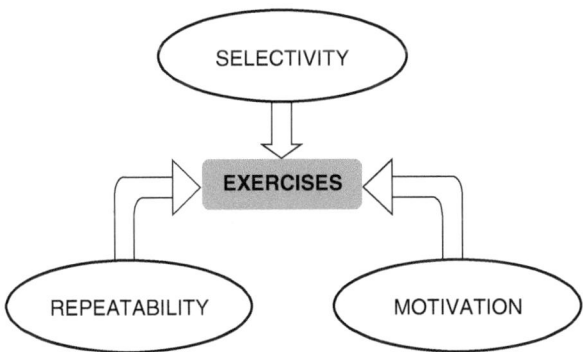

Fig. 3.2 Success criteria for rehabilitation exercises

These two theories could, at least partially, explain the success of integrating games in rehabilitation. Some might think that games are only used in pediatric rehabilitation, it is not the case. Games can be used to increase the quality of rehabilitation for various patients. In order to be effective and to maximize their positive effects, physical rehabilitation exercises must meet three criteria (Fig. 3.2).

We already presented (de)motivation problem, it is obvious that "hiding" rehabilitation exercises within games is a good way to stimulate patients.

Another aspect, closely related to the motivation, is the number of repetitions performed. It has been clearly shown that the more the patient performs repetitions the more gain he will obtain (Langhorne et al. 2011). Since they are focused on the games, patients can perform more repetitions before getting bored when they are playing.

The last point is the selectivity: is the patient performing the right motion? Is there no compensatory or coupled motions? Since the games are goal oriented, patients are somehow guided to perform the right motion.

Despite these, at least potential, positive aspects very little information, or not information at all, can be found in textbook of rehabilitation, on the use of games for children's or adults' rehabilitation (e.g., Dreeben-Irimia 2012; Frontera et al. 2014).

3.3   The Serious Games

3.3.1   Definitions

Thanks to the different, potential, positive aspects of video games presented here above, medical and paramedical field has picked up the positive effects and become interested in the gamification of some medical interventions (Ritterfeld et al. 2009).

Before explaining goals and principles of this new approach, it is important to define the different terms that are used in research and literature.

The term serious games—defined as games designed with a primary purpose other than pure entertainment (healthcare, rehabilitation, education, prevention of injuries, etc.)—is very often used but for some people there is one inadequacy between those two terms, according to them if a game is too serious this is not a game anymore.

On the other hands for some people all games are serious or at least have serious purposes and therefore the term serious games is not an oxymoron (Djaouti et al. 2011). The serious aspect of the games should not take over the fun as nicely explained in this definition *"Games may be played seriously or casually. We are concerned with serious games in the sense that these games have an explicit and carefully thought-out educational purpose and are not intended to be played primarily for amusement. This does not mean that the serious games are not, or should not be, entertaining."* (Abt 1970).

The term serious gaming is used to describe the use of commercial games (e.g., Nintendo Wii™, Microsoft Xbox Kinect) in rehabilitation or in the health care sector.

Personally, I prefer the term exergames (contraction of exercises and games) to describe the use of video games in the revalidation but this term is less used compared to serious games in the literature.

The term virtual reality (VR) is also used but this term is much wider than only performing physical exercises during rehabilitation. The aim of VR is to immerse patient in a virtual environment in order to (re)create some sensory inputs and/or putting patients in various situations that will help him to perform those kinds of activities later on in the real life (Bonnechère et al. 2014). The interactive computer play is one subset of VR-based therapy wherein users can interact with virtual object in a simulated game environment (usually on a two-dimensional screen, not being immersed in 3D virtual environment) and receive real-time feedback on their actions (Ni et al. 2014).

3.3.2 History

It is not obvious to determine when the first serious game was created. According to some authors, it could even be purely entertainment that home video games only appeared after the first digital serious games in the 1970s (Djaouti et al. 2011).

The term serious games, as used today, dates to 2002. Serious games have been developed in various fields. Before 2002, the "ancestors" of serious games were mainly developed for education (66%), advertising (11%), ecology (8%), and healthcare (5%). After 2002, there has been an important decrease in education (26%) and an increase in advertising (31%). The proportion of health care application between 2002 and 2010 represents 8% of the 1265 published studies (Djaouti et al. 2011).

Two famous games popularized the use of serious games in the health care domain and in health prevention. In 1992, the pharmaceutical company Novo Nordisk™ and the video game company Raya System™ developed *"Captain Novolin™"* a game to teach children how to manage diabetes and insulin. The superhero is diabetic and the aim of the game is to control his glucose level. The efficacy of this kind of intervention has been tested in clinical trial. Diabetic children were invited to play *"Packy & Marlon™"* a game similar to the previous one. Compared to a control group, children who play the games managed diabetes better: the number of children who have to go to the hospital due to glucose crisis decreased by 77% in the intervention group (Brown et al. 1997). Currently, this company is a leading publisher of interactive entertainment products designed to promote children's and adolescents' health. Their products are endorsed by the American Academy of Pediatrics, Juvenile Diabetes Foundation, and Asthma and Allergy Foundation of America. The name has been changed into Health Hero Network™ and belongs to the Bosch Healthcare™ group.

Another very popular game that had significant impact on health-related behavior is *"Re-Mission"*. This game was designed for children with cancer in order to teach them how to deal with cancer treatment (mainly chemotherapy) to maximize adherence to treatment. In this game, patients must shoot cancer cells to fight the infections and manage clinical signs and adverse effects (e.g., constipation, nausea).

A clinical trial has been done to compare the effect of *Re-Mission* game and commercial game (Indiana Jones and the Emperor's Tomb™) in adolescents and young adults who were undergoing cancer therapy. Results are shown that patients playing *Re-Mission* significantly improved treatment adherence, indicators of cancer-related self-efficacy, and knowledge.

The findings support current efforts to develop effective video game interventions for education and training in healthcare (Kato et al. 2008). Currently, a second version of the games is freely available on the Internet[5].

3.3.3 Principles of Action

Serious games could be used to assist patients and clinicians in the rehabilitation of various pathologies (see Chap. 4). A common feature, regardless of the approach or the targeted pathology, is that serious games are used, at least partially, to motivate patients to perform their exercises during the rehabilitation process (Tatla et al. 2013).

A group of Canadian researchers has made a lot of work about the motivational aspect of serious gaming for children. The main information of these works have

---

[5] http://www.re-mission2.org/.

been summarized (Miller and Reid 2003; Harris and Reid 2005; Reid 2002, 2004, 2005; Reid and Campbell 2006).

Four points have been identified to improve children's motivation:

1. The key point is the variability of the games. Patients, and more typically children and teenagers, are getting bored of the games. Thus, it's important to have different kinds of games. Even in the same rehabilitation sessions, games must change (e.g., two or three different games for a 1 h session).
2. Finding a good balance in the difficulty levels is an important challenge. It appears that if the game isn't challenging enough, children won't play. On the other hand, if the game is to challenging children will quickly be discouraged and drop out the game.
3. Children are great competitors, thus serious gaming must propose them some competition against robot or other people.
4. The last point is the flexibility of the games. In order to keep the game attractive, patients must be allowed to modify some parameters of the games (speed, number of balls, number of other players, colors, sounds, etc.).

One interesting point of these different works is to try to understand why virtual rehabilitation using serious games is, or could be, efficient. Several theories can be applied to understand the efficacy of serious games:

- Theory of flow (Csikszentmihalyis 1975–1990): The challenges and skills must be equal so the level of serious games must be adapted separately for each patient.
- Motor learning theory (Adams 1981): One of the advantages of serious games is to have a live feedback of the activity. The motor practice combined with live feedback increases motor performance. These benefits must be, in a second time, transferred in activity of daily living.
- Self-efficacy theory (Bandura 1977–1997): It is almost the same point of Adam's theory about transferring performance from game to activity of daily living. If patients improve their performance in real life, and thus their autonomy, they are going to be motivated by the game.

A population of 166 children participated in a study about motivation during rehabilitation. Without surprise the greatest interest is obtained with rewards strategy (for short- and long-term activities) (Gurland and Glowacky 2011).

Although these studies have been performed with children, the same observation and conclusion can be done with adults (Finley and Combs 2013).

3.3.4 Field of Application

The use of serious games in rehabilitation is a relatively new topic; therefore, it is currently difficult to define precisely the field of application and lots of questions still need to be solved such as:

- Which patients could be helped by serious games?
- Which pathology could benefit more from this new approach?
- Which subgroup of patients could respond/not respond to serious games?
- Should the patients play alone at home or only under the supervision of a therapist during the rehabilitation session?
- What is the best frequency? Daily, weekly?
- Are there any adverse effects (fall, seizure)?
- Can the games be counterproductive?

In order to try to answer those questions, the following chapter is presenting the previous works that have been done to test the use of serious games in the treatment of various pathologies.

References

Abt C. Serious games. New-York, USA: Viking Press; 1970.

Adachi PJ, Willoughby T. More than just fun and games: the longitudinal relationships between strategic video games, self-reported problem solving skills, and academic grades. J Youth Adolesc. 2013;42(7):1041–52.

Arvinen-Barrow M, Clement D, Hamson-Utley JJ, Zakrajsek R, Lee S, Kamphoff C, Lintunen T, Hemmings B, Martin S. Athletes' use of mental skills during sport injury rehabilitation. J Sport Rehabil. 2015;24:189–97.

Baer S, Saran K, Green DA. Computer/gaming station use in youth: correlations among use, addiction and functional impairment. Paediatr Child Health. 2012;17(8):427–31.

Baxter RD, Madhok RM. A case of arm swelling and muscle Wii-kness. Scott Med J. 2011;56(4):236.

Bonis J. Acute Wiiitis. N Engl J Med. 2007;356:2431–2.

Bonnechère B, Jansen B, Omelina L, Van Sint Jan S. Integration of exergames and virtual reality in the treatment of cerebral palsy children. In: Yates H, editor. Handbook on cerebral palsy: risk factors, therapeutic management and long-term prognosis. Hauppauge, USA: Nova Science; 2014. p. 25–40. Chap. 2.

Brown SJ, Lieberman DA, Germeny BA, Fan YC, Wilson DM, Pasta DJ. Educational video game for juvenile diabetes: results of a controlled trial. Med Inform (Lond). 1997;22(1):77–89.

Busch V, Manders LA, de Leeuw JR. Screen time associated with health behaviors and outcomes in adolescents. Am J Health Behav. 2013;37(6):819–30.

Cardwell MS. Video media-induced aggressiveness in children. South Med J. 2013;106(9):513–7. Review

Colzato LS, van den Wildenberg WP, Zmigrod S, Hommel B. Action video gaming and cognitive control: playing first person shooter games is associated with improvement in working memory but not action inhibition. Psychol Res. 2013;77(2):234–9.

Costanzo ME, Leaman S, Jovanovic T, Norrholm SD, Rizzo AA, Taylor P, Roy MJ. Psychophysiological response to virtual reality and subthreshold posttraumatic stress disorder symptoms in recently deployed military. Psychosom Med. 2014;76(9):670–7.

Djaouti D, Alvarez J, Jessel JP, Rampnoux O. Origins of serious games. In: Ma M, Oikonomou A, Jain L, editors. Serious games and edutainment applications. London: Springer; 2011. p. 25–43.

Dreeben-Irimia D. Physical therapy clinical handbook for PTAs. 2nd ed. Burlington: MA. Jones & Bartlett Learning; 2012.

Exelmans L, Van den Bulck J. Sleep quality is negatively related to video gaming volume in adults. J Sleep Res. 2015;24(2):189–96.

Ferguson CJ. Violent video games and the supreme court: lessons for the scientific community in the wake of Brown v. Entertainment merchants association. Am Psychol. 2013;68(2):57–74.

Ferguson CJ, Olson CK. Video game violence use among "vulnerable" populations: the impact of violent games on delinquency and bullying among children with clinically elevated depression or attention deficit symptoms. J Youth Adolesc. 2014;43(1):127–36.

Finley M, Combs S. User perceptions of gaming interventions for improving upper extremity motor function in persons with chronic stroke. Physiother Theory Pract. 2013;29(3):195–201.

Frontera WR, Silver JK, Rizzo TD. Essentials of physical medicine and rehabilitation; musculoskeletal disorders, pain and rehabilitation. 3rd ed. Philadelphia, PA: Elsevier Saunders; 2014.

Fullerton S, Taylor AW, Dal Grande E, Berry N. Measuring physical inactivity: do current measures provide an accurate view of "sedentary" videogame time? J Obes. 2014;2014:287013. doi:10.1155/2014/287013. Epub 2014 Jun 4

Galanopoulos I, Garlapati AK, Ashwood N, Kitsis C. A Wii virtual activity severe thumb metacarpal injury. BMJ Case Rep. 2012; 2012. pii: bcr2012006967. doi:10.1136/bcr-2012-006967.

Gates M, Hanning RM, Martin ID, Gates A, Tsuji LJ. Body mass index of first nations youth in Ontario, Canada: influence of sleep and screen time. Rural Remote Health. 2013;13(3):2498.

Gottman JM. The world of coordinated play: same- and cross-sex friendship in young children. Cambridge: Cambridge University Press; 1986.

Granic I, Lobel A, Engels RC. The benefits of playing video games. Am Psychol. 2014;69(1):66–78.

Green CS, Bavelier D. Learning, attentional control, and action video games. Curr Biol. 2012;22(6):R197–206.

Griffiths MD, Davies MN, Chappell D. Online computer gaming: a comparison of adolescent and adult gamers. J Adolesc. 2004;27(1):87–96.

Gurland ST, Glowachy VC. Children's theories of motivation. J Exp Child Psychol. 2011;110(1):1–19.

Harris K, Reid DM. The influence of virtual reality play on children's motivation. Can J Occup Ther. 2005;72(1):21–9.

Hasan Y, Bègue L, Bushman BJ. Violent video games stress people out and make them more aggressive. Aggress Behav. 2013;39(1):64–70.

Hirpara KM, Abouazza OA. The 'Wii knee': a case of patellar dislocation secondary to computer video games. Injury Extra. 2008;38:86–7.

Hoffman AJ. Violent media games and aggression-is it really time for a mea culpa? Am Psychol. 2014;69(3):305–6.

Jalink MB, Heineman E, Pierie JP, Ten Cate Hoedemaker HO. The effect of a preoperative warm-up with a custom-made Nintendo video game on the performance of laparoscopic surgeons. Surg Endosc. 2015;29(8):2284–90.

Kato PM, Cole SW, Bradlyn AS, Pollock BH. A video game improves behavioral outcomes in adolescents and young adults with cancer: a randomized trial. Pediatrics 2008; 122(2): e305–e317.

Khan OA, Parvaiz AC, Vassallo DJ. Acute hernial strangulation following Wii fit exercises. Acta Chir Belg. 2013;113(1):58–9.

Kühn S, Gallinat J. Amount of lifetime video gaming is positively associated with entorhinal, hippocampal and occipital volume. Mol Psychiatry. 2014;19(7):842–7.

Kühn S, Romanowski A, Schilling C, Lorenz R, Mörsen C, Seiferth N, Banaschewski T, Barbot A, Barker GJ, Büchel C, Conrod PJ, Dalley JW, Flor H, Garavan H, Ittermann B, Mann K, Martinot JL, Paus T, Rietschel M, Smolka MN, Ströhle A, Walaszek B, Schumann G, Heinz A, Gallinat J. The neural basis of video gaming. Transl Psychiatry. 2011;1:e53.

Langhorne P, Bernhardt J, Kwakkel G. Stroke rehabilitation. Lancet. 2011;377(9778):1693–702.

Malbos E, Mestre DR, Note ID, Gellato C. Virtual reality and claustrophobia: multiple components therapy involving game editor virtual environments exposure. Cyberpsychol Behav. 2008;11(6):695–7.

Maskey M, Lowry J, Rodgers J, McConachie H, Parr JR. Reducing specific phobia/fear in young people with autism spectrum disorders (ASDs) through a virtual reality environment intervention. PLoS One. 2014;9(7):e100374. doi:10.1371/journal.pone.0100374. eCollection 2014

Melchior M, Chollet A, Fombonne E, Surkan PJ, Dray-Spira R. Internet and video game use in relation to overweight in young adults. Am J Health Promot. 2014;28(4):321–4.

Mellecker RR, Lanningham-Foster L, Levine JA, McManus AM. Energy intake during activity enhanced video game play. Appetite. 2010;55(2):343–7.

Millard HA, Millard RP, Constable PD, Freeman LJ. Relationships among video gaming proficiency and spatial orientation, laparoscopic, and traditional surgical skills of third-year veterinary students. J Am Vet Med Assoc. 2014;244(3):357–62.

Miller S, Reid DT. Doing play: competency, control, and expression. Cyberpsychol Behav. 2003;6(6):623–32.

Ni L, Fehlings D, Biddiss E. Design and evaluation of virtual-reality based therapy games with dual focus on therapeutic relevance and user experience for children with cerebral palsy. Games Health J. 2014;3(3):162–71.

Orbanes P. Monopoly: the World's most Famous Game & how it got that way. Cambridge: Da Capo Press; 2006.

Peek AC, Ibrahim T, Abunasra H, Waller D, Natarajan R. White-out from a Wii: traumatic haemothorax sustained playing Nintendo Wii. Ann R Coll Surg. 2008;90:9–10.

Piaget J. Play, dreams and imitation. New York: Norton; 1962.

Razavi H, Lam G. Wii eye injury: self-inflicted globe rupture and vision loss in a 7-year-old boy from a video game accident. J AAPOS. 2011;15(5):491–2.

Reid DT. Virtutal reality and the person-environment experience. Cyberpsychol Behav. 2002;5(6):559–64.

Reid DT. The influence of virtual reality on playfulness in children with cerebral palsy: a pilot study. Occup Ther Int. 2004;11(3):131–44.

Reid DT. Correlation of the pediatric volitional questionnaire with the test of playfulness in a virtual environment: the power of engagement. Early Child Dev Care. 2005;175(2):153–64.

Reid D, Campbell K. The use of virtual reality with children with cerebral palsy: a pilot randomized trial. Ther Recreat J. 2006;40(4):255–68.

Ritterfeld U, Cody M, Vorderer P, editors. Serious games: mechanisms and effects. New York: Taylor & Francis; 2009.

Rothbaum BO, Price M, Jovanovic T, Norrholm SD, Gerardi M, Dunlop B, Davis M, Bradley B, Duncan EJ, Rizzo A, Ressler KJ. A randomized, double-blind evaluation of D-cycloserine or alprazolam combined with virtual reality exposure therapy for posttraumatic stress disorder in Iraq and Afghanistan war veterans. Am J Psychiatry. 2014;171(6):640–8.

Rus-Calafell M, Gutiérrez-Maldonado J, Botella C, Baños RM. Virtual reality exposure and imaginal exposure in the treatment of fear of flying: a pilot study. Behav Modif. 2013;37(4):568–90.

Siervo M, Sabatini S, Fewtrell MS, Wells JC. Acute effects of violent video-game playing on blood pressure and appetite perception in normal-weight young men: a randomized controlled trial. Eur J Clin Nutr. 2013;67(12):1322–4.

Spinks AB, Macpherson AK, Bain C, McClure RJ. Compliance with the Australian national physical ctivity guidelines for children: relationship to overweight status. J Sci Med Sport. 2007;10(3):156–63.

Tatla SK, Sauve K, Virji-Babul N, Holsti L, Butler C, Van Der Loos HF. Evidence for outcomes of motivational rehabilitation interventions for children and adolescents with cerebral palsy: an American Academy for Cerebral Palsy and Developmental Medicine systematic review. Dev Med Child Neurol. 2013;55(7):593–601.

Tear MJ, Nielsen M. Failure to demonstrate that playing violent video games diminishes prosocial behavior. PLoS One. 2013;8(7):e68382.

Weaver JB 3rd, Mays D, Sargent Weaver S, Kannenberg W, Hopkins GL, Eroğlu D, Bernhardt JM. Health-risk correlates of video-game playing among adults. Am J Prev Med. 2009;37(4):299–305.

Wells JJ. An 8-year-old girl presented to the ER after accidentally being hit by a Wii remote control swung by her brother. J Trauma. 2008;65:1203.

West GL, Al-Aidroos N, Pratt J. Action video game experience affects oculomotor performance. Acta Psychol. 2013;142(1):38–42.

Whitbourne SK, Ellenberg S, Akimoto K. Reasons for playing casual video games and perceived benefits among adults 18 to 80 years old. Cyberpsychol Behav Soc Netw. 2013;16(12):892–7.

White K, Schofield G, Kilding AE. Energy expended by boys playing active video games. J Sci Med Sport. 2011;14(2):130–4.

Willis RE, Gomez PP, Ivatury SJ, Mitra HS, Van Sickle KR. Virtual reality simulators: valuable surgical skills trainers or video games? J Surg Educ. 2014;71(3):426–33.

World Health Organization (WHO). Global recommendations on physical activity for health. Geneva: World Health Organization; 2010.

Serious Games in Rehabilitation

4

Over the years, our patients have shared some amazing and emotional stories as they've recovered from an injury, illness, or surgery which required some degree of physical rehabilitation. For many of our patients, once they've experienced a disability, they work with unwavering strength and courage to return to the lifestyle of their choosing. Their stories are compelling and emphasize the perseverance of the human spirit. In sharing their experiences, our former patients are reminded of their own strength, and are benefiting those who are now in a similar situation. Reading these stories will hopefully provide inspiration to those who are at the beginning of their own physical rehabilitation process and others who are not sure what physical rehabilitation is all about.

– Kathleen Yosko

4.1 General Discussion

The results presented in this chapter covered the work published in the field until end 2015 (meta-analysis). A systematic search was conducted to identify empirical studies that evaluated the effectiveness of commercial video games in physical rehabilitation programs (Bonnechère et al. 2016). Same methodology was used for serious games (specially developed games for physical rehabilitation).

Medline, SAGE journals online, and Science Direct databases were screened using a combination of the following free-text terms: commercial games, video games, exergames, serious gaming, serious games, rehabilitation games, PlayStation, Nintendo, Wii, Wii Fit, Xbox, and Kinect. The search was limited to peer-reviewed English journals. There beginning of the search time frame was not restricted because this is a fairly recent paradigm; the search time frame ended on December 31, 2015.

Before discussing the use of serious games from a medical points of view: advantages, limitations, risks, etc.—let's have a look on the general use of the games in physical rehabilitation.

© Springer International Publishing AG 2018
B. Bonnechère, *Serious Games in Physical Rehabilitation*,
https://doi.org/10.1007/978-3-319-66122-3_4

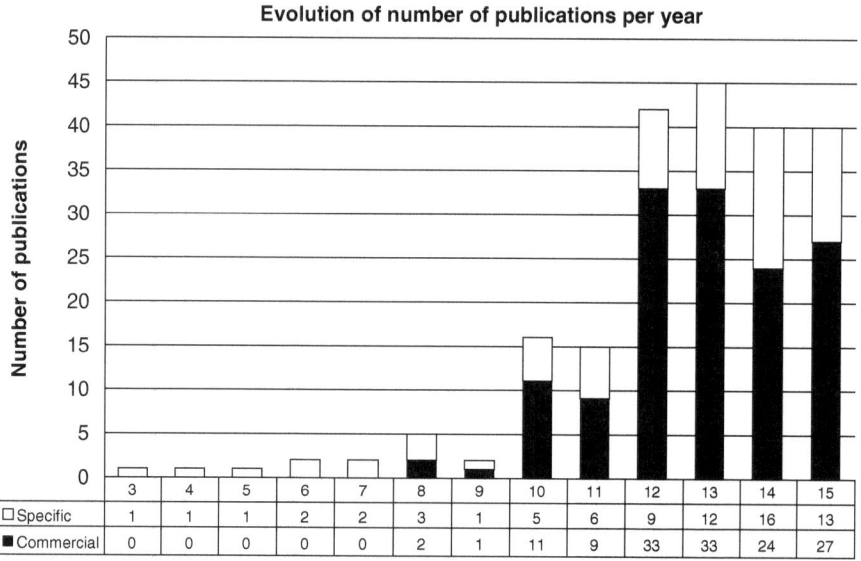

Fig. 4.1 Number of publications about the use of video games in rehabilitation per year

4.1.1 A New Trend?

We already discussed and presented the development of computer and technologies related to the games in the last decades (see Chap. 1). Therefore, it is not surprising to observe an important increase of the number of studies and publications since 2010 (the Wii was released in 2007 and the Kinect sensor in 2010). Before the commercialization of those popular commercial devices, the creation of serious games required development of both hardware and software.

Thanks to the large availability, and affordable price, of the sensors developed by and for gaming purposes, researchers and developers can easily develop specific games and solution for physical rehabilitation.

Since 2010, approximately one third of the tested games are specially developed exergames (Fig. 4.1).

4.1.2 Commercial or Specific Games?

Figure 4.1 presents the use of commercial (black) and specific games (white). 212 studies were included in this review. The repartition is two third about commercial video games (140 studies) and one third for specific solutions (72 studies). From a theoretical point of view both systems have advantages and disadvantages that are summarized in Table 4.1.

Table 4.1 Advantages and disadvantages of commercial and specific games for rehabilitation

	Commercial games	Specific games
Motions to perform	• Based on speed • Maximal range of motions	• Configurable (speed, range of motion, etc.)
Rehabilitation	• Not based on rehabilitation schemes	• Designed for a particular rehabilitation purpose (balance, strength, coordination, dexterity, etc.)
Safety	• Risk of fall: difficult to estimate due to lack of existing date in the literature	• Risk of fall: difficult to estimate due to lack of existing date in the literature. However, since games are designed for rehabilitation it can be expected that this risk is lower since the motions that need to be performed by the patients are similar to those performed during rehabilitation
Availability	• Worldwide • Large distribution • Advertising and marketing	• Specialized center • Internet
Price	• Cheap	• In general, more expensive (market size)
Usability	• Very large number of users • User friendly • Stable	• "Niche" market • More complex but closer to the clinics and rehabilitation
Marketing	• Directly to customer (B2C)	• Clinicians are selling or renting the product (B2B)

Table 4.2 Number of studies and patients' repartition among the selected studies

	Commercial games		Specific games		Total	
	Studies	Patients	Studies	Patients	Studies	Patients
Aging	41	1353	10	907	51	2260
Obesity	13	1094	9	867	22	1961
Stroke	35	766	18	724	53	1490
Balance	26	926	16	379	42	1305
CP	16	339	15	315	31	654
PD	9	170	4	68	13	238
Total	140	4648	72	3260	212	7908

4.1.3 For Which Patients?

Six main pathologies/conditions were discussed individually because there were enough studies in the literature in this field: aging, obesity and weight management, stroke, balance impairment, cerebral palsy (CP), and Parkinson's disease (PD). The repartitions of the patients included in those studies are presented in Tables 4.2 and 4.3.

Table 4.3 Mean duration (session) of the studies by pathology

	Commercial games	Specific games	Total
Aging	20 (8)	21 (15)	20
Obesity	59 (36)	43 (23)	52
Stroke	16 (10)	13 (6)	14
Balance	19 (9)	14 (11)	16
CP	23 (18)	18 (16)	20
PD	16 (6)	14 (11)	15
Total	25	21	

Fig. 4.2 Patients' repartition for commercial games

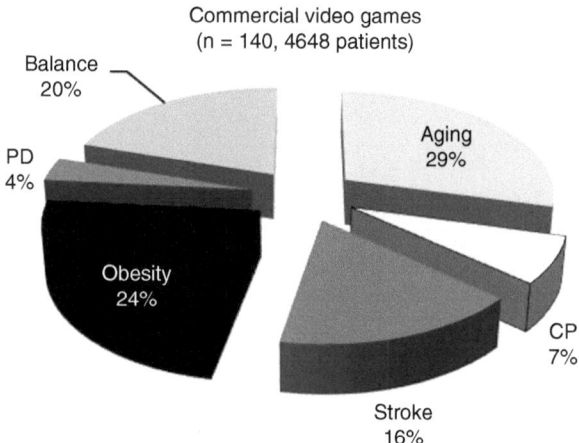

Commercial video games
(n = 140, 4648 patients)

Balance 20%
PD 4%
Obesity 24%
Aging 29%
CP 7%
Stroke 16%

Although there is almost the same number of studies about aging, for stroke rehabilitation the number of patients included is much more important for aging. The second most studied population are obese and overweighed subjects. Those numbers are relatively coherent and reflect the prevalence of these conditions/pathologies (see Table 7.1).

The repartition of the patients in the different studies between commercial and specific games is presented in Table 4.2, in Fig. 4.2 for commercial video games, in Fig. 4.3 for specific games, and for both approaches in Fig. 4.4.

4.1.4 Number of Session?

Depending on the pathologies, and the severity of the disease, the duration of the rehabilitation varies a lot. Except for the management of obesity that required longer intervention for the other pathologies the mean duration is approximately 18 sessions which correspond more or less to the duration of the conventional rehabilitation treatment.

Fig. 4.3 Patients'
repartition for specific
games

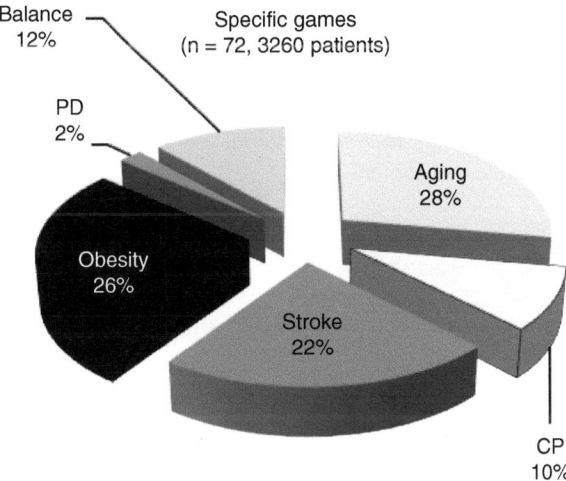

Fig. 4.4 Patients divided
by pathology

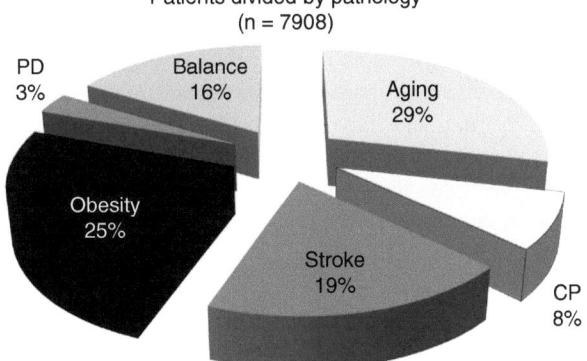

4.2 Aging

4.2.1 Clinical Presentation

Of course, aging is not a pathology by itself but aging is associated with physiological decline of various systems and functions.

The two main problems related to the elderly are: a significant increase of risk of fall and a natural decline of cognitive functions.

Since the population of developed countries is getting older, a lot of efforts are done and must be done to improve autonomy and decreased risk of fall. A dramatic statistic illustrates the importance of avoiding falls: the most common fractures in case of fall are wrist and femoral neck. In case of femoral neck fracture, the mortality rate after 1, 6, 12, and 24 months are 5%, 16%, 21%, and 30%, respectively (Meessen et al. 2014). Hip fracture incidence per 1000 persons of above 70 years old is 8.4 in women and 3.7 in men (Meessen et al. 2014).

Therefore, decreasing risk of fall and cognitive decline of the elderly is a major health care problem.

4.2.2   Rehabilitation

In order to prevent risk of falls, different approaches are possible in physiotherapy and rehabilitation: to increase coordination between legs, to increase the proprioception (i.e., sense of relative position of joints in space), to maintain "normal," or at least functional, range of motion of the most important joints (e.g., hip and knee).

Dual-task training is another popular approach in physiotherapy to decrease risk of falls. Dual-task training consists in performing simultaneously two tasks—often a motor task and a cognitive task: the best-known case is to ask the patient to walk while counting.

Occupational therapists have also an important role to modify the living environment in order to be as safe as possible (e.g., avoid carpet, sufficient lights).

The vision, in particular the visual field, must also be checked since a lot of elderly patients have a visual field loss (i.e., scotoma due to macular degeneration).

Concerning the cognitive function, it appears that the best way to prevent cognitive decline is to train your brain and memory (reading, exercises, games), the famous quote *"use it or lose it"* is particularly true in this field.

4.2.3   Use of Serious Games

4.2.3.1 Musculoskeletal Rehabilitation

Summary of the different studies included are presented in Tables 4.4 and 4.5 for commercial video games and specific ones, respectively. 51 studies were found in the literature. Repartitions of devices and approaches are presented in Fig. 4.5.

Most of these studies (72%) were done using commercial video games and especially the Nintendo Wii combined with the Balance Board (20 studies). We observed that the games were mainly used to increase balance and postural control. Results of these studies indicate that results obtained with video games are at least as good as the results obtained with traditional balance exercises for balance and reaching area (e.g., Agmon et al. 2011, Rendon et al. 2012, Bieryla and Dold 2013, Cho et al. 2014, Roopchand-Martin et al. 2015).

Sarcopenia is the degenerative loss of skeletal muscle mass, quality, and strength associated with aging. Sarcopenia is one of the main causes of the decrease of autonomy of elderly subjects and one of the factors responsible for the increased risk of fall. Two studies have shown significant improvement for maximal leg

Table 4.4 Summary of studies about commercial video games included in this review on aging for musculoskeletal rehabilitation

Study and Year	Device	Subjects	Interventions	Outcomes
Nacke et al. (2009)	Nintendo Wii	21 older adults	1 session of play comparing brain training™ and traditional calculation on paper sheets	The delivery of those VG training in digital form does not improve players' effectiveness or efficiency, regardless of age. However, the VG form does make the tasks more exciting and induces a heightened sense of flow in gamers of all ages
Guderian et al. (2010)	Nintendo Wii	20 older adults	1 session of 20 min of games (6 separate aerobic and balance games).	Results indicate that playing VG is a feasible alternative to more traditional aerobic exercise modalities for middle-aged and older adults
Ackerman et al. (2010)	Nintendo Wii	78 older adults	4 weeks of training, 5 session a day, followed by 4 weeks of 4 weeks of reading (5 sessions a day)	Improvements on the Wii tasks, less improvement on the domain-knowledge tests, and practice-related improvements. No significant transfer-of-training from either the VG or the reading tasks to measures of cognitive abilities.
Rosenberg et al. (2010)	Nintendo Wii	19 community-dwelling adults	12 weeks of training, 3 sessions per week	Significant improvement in depressive symptoms, mental health-related quality of life, and cognitive performance, but not physical health-related quality of life.
Graves et al. (2010)	Nintendo Wii	42 participants (14 adolescents, 15 young adults, and 13 older adults)	1 session of games comparing inactive video gaming, active video gaming, and brisk treadmill walking and jogging	Heart rates and energy expenditure during VG aerobics exercises fell below the recommended intensity for maintaining cardiorespiratory fitness. Group enjoyment rating was greater for VG balance and aerobics compared with treadmill walking and jogging
Williams et al. (2010)	Nintendo Wii	21 community-dwelling fallers separated into interventions or conventional treatment group	12 weeks of training, 2 sessions per week	VG exercise is acceptable in self-referred older people with a history of falls. The games have the potential to improve balance

(continued)

Table 4.4 (continued)

Study and Year	Device	Subjects	Interventions	Outcomes
Ackerman et al. (2010)	Nintendo Wii	78 older adults	4 weeks of training, 5 sessions per week	Significant improvements during VG, but no significant transfer from either the VG or reading tasks to measures of cognitive and perceptual speed
Agmon et al. (2011)	Nintendo Wii	7 older adults	12 weeks of training, 3 sessions per week	Significant improve in the Berg Balance Score and in walking speed after intervention
Laver et al. (2011)	Nintendo Wii	21 older adults	5 sessions per week for the duration of patient stay	Following the therapy program, participants were more concerned with the mode of therapy and preferred traditional therapy programs over programs using the VG.
Lamoth et al. (2011)	Nintendo Wii	9 older adults	6 weeks of training, 3 sessions per week	Postural control improved during the intervention. After the intervention, period task performance and balance were better than before the intervention
Williams et al. (2011)	Nintendo Wii	22 community living older adults	4 weeks of training, 3 sessions per week	Significant improvement in balance after intervention
Hsu et al. (2011)	Nintendo Wii	34 older adults separated into intervention and standard exercises group	4 weeks of training and 4 weeks of standard exercises (crossing over)	Significant improvement for pain intensity, physical activity for both groups. Enjoyment level was higher is the intervention group
Bateni (2012)	Nintendo Wii	12 older adults separated in 3 groups: Physical therapy alone, games alone, or both games and therapy	4 weeks of training, 3 sessions per week	VG training appears to improve balance. However, physical therapy training on its own or in addition to games training appears to improve balance to a greater extent than VG alone
Daniel (2012)	Nintendo Wii	Older adults separated in 3 groups: Fitness classes, intervention, and control group (no intervention)	15 weeks of training, 2 sessions per week	Similar results for the intervention group compared to community-based senior fitness classes
Rendon et al. (2012)	Nintendo Wii	40 older adults separated in intervention or control group	6 weeks of training, 3 sessions per week	Significant improvement for balance and postural stability in the intervention group

Study	Platform	Participants	Training	Results
Griffin et al. (2012)	Nintendo Wii	65 older adults separated into intervention and conventional balance therapy group	7 weeks of training	Significant improvement for both groups. Significant greater improvement in the intervention group. VG can provide an effective adjunct to standard rehabilitation
Franco et al. (2012)	Nintendo Wii	32 independent living senior separated in 3 groups: Intervention group, conventional balance program, and control group (no intervention)	3 weeks of training, 2 sessions per week	No statistical significant difference was found between the 3 groups (the duration of the intervention may have been too short)
Pluchino et al. (2012)	Nintendo Wii	40 elderly separated into intervention and conventional therapy group	8 weeks of training, 2 sessions per week	VG are as effective as standard balance exercises program
Toulotte et al. (2012)	Nintendo Wii	36 older adults separated in 4 groups: Adapted physical activities, intervention group, combined, and no intervention group	20 weeks of training, 1 session per week	The three intervention groups improved their balance. Adapted physical activities and combined group also improved dynamic balance
Padala et al. (2012)	Nintendo Wii	22 subjects with mild Alzheimer's dementia separated into intervention program and walking program	8 weeks of training, 5 sessions per week	No difference was found between group. Use of VG resulted in significant improvements in balance and gait compared to those in the robust monitored walking program
Orsega-Smith et al. (2012)	Nintendo Wii	25 overweight older adults	8 weeks of training, 2 sessions per week	Significant improvement in balance, confidence, and activities of daily living
Chan et al. (2012)	Nintendo Wii	30 older adults from geriatric day hospital	8 sessions of training included into conventional rehabilitation program	VG can be used in geriatric day hospital, most participants accepted it and had more improvement in functional independent measure compared to conventional rehabilitation

(continued)

Table 4.4 (continued)

Study and Year	Device	Subjects	Interventions	Outcomes
Taylor et al. (2012)	Nintendo Wii and Xbox Kinect	19 community-dwelling	1 single session of play. 9 different games were tested in both sitting or standing position	No significant difference in energy expenditure, activity counts, or perceived exertion between equivalent games played while standing and sitting. Active video games provide light-intensity exercise in community-dwelling older people, whether played while sitting or standing
Kim et al. (2013)	Xbox Kinect	32 ambulatory older adults separated into intervention and control group	8 weeks of training, 3 sessions per week	The VG exercise program includes the role of supervisor and feedback, which is important for older adults. Therefore, a VR-based exercise program may be a useful tool to improve decreased physical function in older adults as a home-based exercise
Singh et al. (2013)	Nintendo Wii	36 community-dwelling older women separated into virtual reality balance group and conventional balance exercises	6 weeks of training, 2 sessions per week	No significant differences between groups, both group improved balance and functional mobility score
Chao et al. (2013)	Nintendo Wii	7 older adults	8 weeks of training, 2 sessions per week	Participants had significant improvement on balance. Although not significant differences, there were trends indicating that participants improved mobility, walking endurance, and decreased fear of falling
Jorgensen et al. (2013)	Nintendo Wii	58 community living older adults separate into intervention group and control group (daily use of ethylene vinyl acetate copolymer insoles)	10 weeks of training, 2 sessions per week	Significant improvement in maximal leg muscle strength and overall functional performance in the intervention group. No difference on balance between groups

Study	Platform	Participants	Training	Results
Bieryla et al. (2013)	Nintendo Wii	12 healthy older adults separated into interventions and control group	3 weeks of training, 3 sessions per week	Significant increase in the Berg Balance Scale in the intervention group, no significant change for Fullerton Advanced Balance scale, functional reach or timed up and go
Keogh et al. (2013)	Nintendo Wii	34 older adults separated into interventions and control group	8 weeks of training, 3 sessions per week	Significant increase in muscular endurance, physical activity levels and psychological quality of life in the intervention group
Lee et al. (2013)	PlayStation 2	55 older adults with diabetes mellitus separated into interventions and control group	10 weeks of training, 2 sessions per week.	Significant improvement in balance, gait speed, cadence and falls efficacy, decreased sit-to-stand times in the intervention group
Cho et al. (2014)	Nintendo Wii	32 healthy adults separated into interventions and control group	8 weeks of training, 3 sessions per week	Significant improvement in the VG games compared to control group. VG training can be proposed as a form of fall prevention exercise for the elderly
Maillot et al. (2014)	Nintendo Wii	67 participants (32 young and 32 old adults).	12 weeks of training, 2 sessions per week	VG appears to be an effective way to train postural control in older adults. Because of the multimodal nature of the activity, exergames provide an effective tool for remediation of age-related problems
Jung et al. (2015)	Nintendo Wii	24 older adults	8 weeks of training, 2 sessions per week	Significant improvements in obstacle negotiation function after VG compared to the control group. Berg Balance Scale and functional reach test scores were greater in the lumbar stabilization exercise group, while timed up-and-go test time was significantly better in the VG group
Monteiro-Junior et al. (2015)	Nintendo Wii	30 older women with chronic low back pain	8 weeks of training, 3 sessions per week	Capacity to sit only improved in the VG group, significant decrease in pain, but no balance improvements

(continued)

Table 4.4 (continued)

Study and Year	Device	Subjects	Interventions	Outcomes
Fu et al. (2015)	Nintendo Wii	60 older adults	6 weeks of training, 3 sessions per week	Physiological profile assessment scores and incidence of falls improved significantly in both groups after the intervention, but participants in the VG group showed significantly greater improvement in both outcome measures
Nicholson et al. (2015)	Nintendo Wii	41 older adults	6 weeks of training, 3 sessions per week	Significant improvements in timed up-and-go, left single-leg balance, lateral reach (left and right), and gait speed
Chao et al. (2015)	Nintendo Wii	32 older adults	4 weeks of training, 2 sessions per week	Significant improvements in balance, mobility, and depression
Roopchand-Martin et al. (2015)	Nintendo Wii	28 older adults	6 weeks training, 2 sessions per week	Significant improvement in balance and reaching area. No significant change on the modified clinical test for sensory integration in balance
Höchsmann et al. (2016)	Nintendo Wii	12 diabetic older patients	1 session	VG offers training intensities that are consistent with established guidelines for older patients with type 2 diabetes
Karahan et al. (2015)	Xbox Kinect	100 older adults	6 weeks of training, 5 sessions per week	Significant improvement in balance, quality of life parameters of physical functioning, social role functioning, physical role restriction, and general health perception

Table 4.5 Summary of studies about specific rehabilitation games included in this review on aging for musculoskeletal rehabilitation

Study and Year	Subjects	Interventions	Outcomes
Szturm et al. (2014)	30 community-dwelling older subjects separated into interventions and control group	8 weeks of training, 2 sessions per week of computer games	Dynamic balance exercises on fixed and compliant sponge surfaces were feasibly coupled to interactive game-based exercise. This coupling, in turn, resulted in a greater improvement in dynamic standing balance control compared with the typical exercise program
Chen et al. (2012a, b)	40 community-dwelling older subjects separated into interventions and control group	6 weeks of training, 2 sessions per week of balance training	For clinical assessments (balance, mobility, and self-confidence), SG group showed significantly better scores. The movements in video game-based training mimic real-life situations which may help to transfer the training effects into daily activities
Lai et al. (2013)	30 community-living older subjects separated into interventions and control group	6 weeks of training, 3 sessions per week	SG training improves balance after 6 weeks of implementation, and the beneficial effects partially remain after training is complete
Duque et al. (2013)	60 community-dwelling older subjects separated into interventions and control group	6 weeks of training, 2 sessions per week of balance training	Balance parameters were significantly improved in the SG group. This effect was also associated with a significant reduction in falls and lower levels of fear of falling
Schoene et al. (2013)	37 older adults in independent-living units	8 weeks of training, 2–3 sessions per week of balance training	Step pad training can be safely undertaken at home to improve physical and cognitive parameters of fall risk in older people without major cognitive and physical impairments
Uzor et al. (2013)	48 older adults at risk of falling separated into interventions and control group	12 weeks of training age UK falls rehabilitation booklet (home-based rehabilitation exercises)	It is a feasibility study. The presented system seems to be a feasible tool for fall preventions at home
Gschwind et al. (2014)	160 community-dwelling older people	16 weeks of training, 180 min per week of balance training	It is a feasibility study. The presented system seems to be a feasible tool for fall preventions at home

(continued)

Table 4.5 (continued)

Study and Year	Subjects	Interventions	Outcomes
Schwenk et al. (2014)	33 older adults with fall risk separate into interventions and control group	4 weeks of training, 2 sessions per weeks	Improvement was obtained for timed up-and-go test, fast gait speed, but not normal gait speed. Users expressed a positive training experience of sensor-feedback
Gschwind et al. (2015)	148 community dwelling people	16 weeks of training, 180 min per week of balance training	Compared to the control group, VG participants improved their fall risk score, proprioception, reaction time, sit-to-stand performance, and executive functioning

Fig. 4.5 Repartition of the devices for studies on aging for musculoskeletal rehabilitation

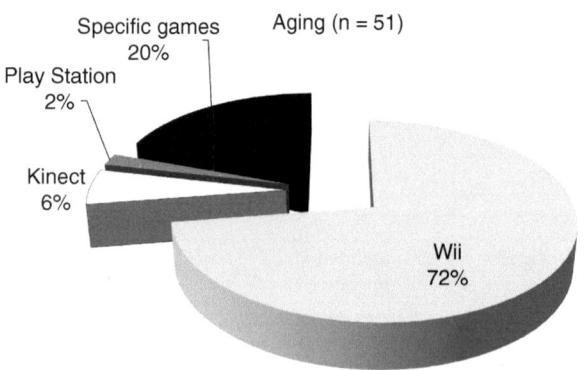

strength after 10 weeks of training (Jorgensen et al. 2013) and for muscular endurance after 8 weeks of training (Keogh et al. 2013).

It is interesting to note that the games are well accepted by the participants even though they are, usually, unaccustomed to video games. Elderly subjects accept to use this technology (the level of participation is high). The level of enjoyment during rehabilitation exercises performed with the games in higher compared to traditional balance exercises; therefore, those kinds of games could be used to motivate patients and increase the participation during the rehabilitation process (Nacke et al. 2009).

Another positive point is that playing games seems to increase subjects' confidence during activity of daily living and decrease the fear of falling and the kinesiophobia (Orsega-Smith et al. 2012).

One last interesting point is that playing video games is a feasible alternative to more traditional aerobic exercises for older adults (Guderian et al. 2010). However, it is obvious that playing games does not equal the treadmill training, walking or jogging, and therefore video games training does not totally fulfill the requirement to maintain cardiorespiratory fitness in the elderly (Graves et al. 2010).

However for some specific patients and pathologies (e.g., diabetic older patients), the training intensity reached during the serious games are consistent with the established guidelines (Höchsmann et al. 2016). Therefore, the games could be an interesting alternative since patients seem to prefer to use VG for balance or aerobics training.

Since commercial video games are not designed for rehabilitation, the transfer between progresses in the games and during activities of daily living and/or the therapeutic relevance of such kind of approach may be challenged by some clinicians.

In order to be more specific and close to the clinics, rehabilitation games have been specially developed for elderly subjects. Significant improvements have been found for balance (Lai et al. 2013) and decreasing the risk of fall (Duque et al. 2013).

A set of specific games have been developed to train real-life situation (obstacle avoidance, transfer from sitting to standing, etc.), after 6 weeks of training researchers found significant improvement in balance, mobility, and self-confidence but also significant improvement during activities of daily livings (Chen et al. 2012b). This study, and other works related to the integration of specific rehabilitation games within conventional treatment, underlines the importance of goal-oriented training to increase transfert between rehabilitation session at the clinic and activities of daily living.

4.2.3.2 Cognitive Training

Although this book is about the physical rehabilitation, the problem related to cognitive decline is such an important health issue that we are going to discuss briefly the use of games for cognitive training of the elderly.

One meta-analysis has been published that summarized previous works performed in the field of cognitive training for elderly patients using video games. Twenty studies have been included in this study (only studies with a control group to compare the results of the intervention) (Toril et al. 2014). Results of the studies indicate that the games have a positive effect on different cognitive functions such as reaction time, attention, and memory. The authors conclude that the use of video games can be used to counter the natural age-related decline of cognitive function. However, further studies are still needed to determine which kind of intervention (type of games, number of games, number of sessions) is the best and which kind of personal factors (genetics, environment, education) may influence the results.

It has been shown that the progress in the games (and therefore in cognitive function) are directly correlated to the age of the participants and the number of session of gaming. It is now well accepted that cognitive video games have a positive impact on brain function with the elderly but there is still no consensus in the literature about the best use of these games.

A lot of questions still need to be answered. What is the influence of age of the learning effect? What is the best kind of games? What is the best duration of intervention?

A last interesting point has been highlighted over the last years. The learning capacity would not be affected by the cognitive decline. It is still possible to learn regardless age or cognitive level. Therefore, the same kind of benefice could be reached by elderly and by adults after a cognitive intervention program (Anguera et al. 2013, Bamidis et al. 2015).

4.3   Obesity and Overweight

4.3.1   Clinical Presentation

Obesity by itself is not a pathology but is a very important health-related problem that can lead to several pathologies such as hypertension, and hypercholesterolemia and therefore drastically increase the risk of stroke, myocardial infarction, diabetes, cancers, etc. Recent studies also demonstrated a link between obesity and Alzheimer's disease probably due to the accumulation of fat tissues and the role of fat tissue on the hormonal system.

Overweight and obesity are defined as abnormal or excessive fat accumulation in the body that presents a risk to health. Simple indicator of obesity is the body mass index (BMI) that is equal to the weight (in kilograms) divided by the square of the height (in meters). A person with a BMI of 30 or more is considered obese. A person with a BMI equal to or more than 25 is considered overweight (WHO).

Obesity is a huge health care problem in the world; according to the WHO, it is estimated that 12% of the people (aged 20 and over) are obese and 35% are overweight[1]. Obesity is not any more a problem related to high-income countries; the prevalence of obesity and overweight exploding in emerging countries (Table 7.1) presents the prevalence of obesity in different region of the world.

In some particular cases (2–3%), obesity is caused by endocrinal troubles (hypothyroidism, adrenal gland disease), but in most cases, it is caused by an excess of energy intake and insufficient energy expenditure (exercises).

4.3.2   Rehabilitation

Management of obesity and overweight problem is complex and requires a multi-disciplinary team: nutritionist and food specialists to modify food habits, psychologists to modify body image and perception of the body, physiotherapists to promote physical activities, and medical doctors to control the associated disorders.

The aim of rehabilitation is obvious with obese patients: patients need to move in order to burn calories, physical activity also stimulates these patients and improves proprioception, the perception of the body, and increases self-esteem.

The power and strength of the group should also be considered in physical rehabilitation. It is important for the patients to work together, share their difficulties, and visualize their progresses. Group session are organized under the supervision of

---

[1] http://www.who.int/gho/ncd/risk_factors/overweight/en/index.html

a multidisciplinary team to help those patients. Group therapy is also commonly proposed for patients suffering from low back pain, fibromyalgia, multiple sclerosis, cancers, etc.

4.3.3 Use of Serious Games

Obesity problem has been, partly, addressed by the industry of commercial video games since a lot of fitness games have been developed in order to make patients more active. Specific games have been created to develop fitness skills (e.g., Nintendo Wii Fit™) and thanks to the development of new way of controlling the games (mainly Nintendo Wii™ and Microsoft Xbox Kinect™) the energy expenditure have been increasing when playing video games (see Sect. 3.1.2.2).

Summary of the different studies included are presented in Tables 4.6 and 4.7 for commercial video games and specific ones, respectively. 22 studies were found in the literature. Repartitions of devices and approaches are presented in Fig. 4.6.

It is interesting to note that 40% solutions are specific games. Actually in this case, it is more accurate to speak of teaching and monitoring programs (in most cases via the Internet) for controlling and modifying eating behavior rather than developing solutions to make the patients more active (e.g., Wagener et al. 2012; Christison and Khan 2012).

The first question to answer is whether or not the active video games induce an increase of energy expenditure and if yes what is the level of physical activity reached during this kind of training. Many studies have been conducted in this field.

The level of energy expenditure reached is estimated between 2.7 and 5.4 metabolic equivalents (i.e., moderate intensity level of physical activity) when children and teenagers play active games. A study compared the levels of energy expenditure in an obese population and in a control group, surprisingly the author found that obese children burnt fewer calories than the control group (O'Donovan et al. 2014).

We already mentioned that playing active video games correspond to the same energy expenditure level as the level reached during walking and are therefore not enough to fulfill WHO recommendation (60 min per day of moderate physical activity) (White et al. 2011). Another study compared the energy expended during a fitness game and a balance game. 100 people, including 55 overweight people, participated in this study. The same levels of physical activity were found when playing the fitness game (still below the WHO recommendations) that in previous studies but lower energy expenditure for balance games but the patients preferred to play balance games instead of fitness games (Lyons et al. 2012).

Although we saw that the levels of energy expenditure reached are relatively low, could these games still be successfully integrated into the management of obesity and overweight?

The first large study was conducted in 2012, 171 obese students were included. They were separated into two groups: 63 people were included in the group playing video games and the other 108 in a control group. After 9 weeks of training, the level of physical activity was higher in the intervention group and patients had lost

Table 4.6 Summary of studies about commercial video games included in this review on obesity and overweight

Study and Year	Device	Subjects	Interventions	Outcomes
Graves et al. (2010)	PlayStation 2	44 children	12 weeks of training	No significant body fat changes between groups
Maddison et al. (2011)	PlayStation 2	322 young adults	Active video games or sedentary video games (control)	BMI intervention no change, increase of BMI in control, decrease of body fat in intervention. Time playing active video games increase with decrease in time playing no active video games
Lyons et al. (2012)	Nintendo Wii	100 young adults (55 overweight)	1 session of games: 1 aerobic and 1 balance game	Aerobic games produced more energy that balance game but balance games are more enjoyable
Johnston et al. (2012)	Nintendo Wii	63 students in the interventions group and 108 controls	9 weeks of games	Physical activity level was significantly increased in the VG group and participants lost 1.5 to 2 kg after the intervention
Staiano et al. (2012a, b)	Nintendo Wii	31 low-income overweight or obese adolescent separate into competitive exergames or cooperative exergames	6 months of training, 5 sessions per week	Cooperative exergames play produced higher intrinsic motivation. Players with higher intrinsic motivation had higher energy expenditure
Staiano et al. (2012a, b)	Nintendo Wii	74 overweight students	26 sessions over 20 weeks	Significant weight reduction
Feltz et al. (2012)	PlayStation 2	135 students separate into 4 different experimental conditions	1 session of games under different conditions: (individual control or low-, moderate-, or high-partner discrepancy)	Virtually presented partners who are moderately more capable than participants are the most effective at improving persistence in VG

Quinn (2013)	Nintendo Wii	86 obese students	VG was incorporated into physical education class to increase student participation	Children were more active after interventions
Staiano et al. (2013)	Nintendo Wii	54 overweight or obese adolescent separate into cooperative, competitive exergames, or control group	20 weeks of training, 5 sessions a week	Cooperative exergame players lost significantly more weight than the control group and the competitive group, which did not lose weight
Tripette et al. (2014)	Nintendo Wii	34 postpartum women separate into intervention, or control group	40 days of training	Statistically significant reductions of BMI, waist and hip circumference, and body fat
Trost et al. (2014)	Xbox Kinect	75 overweight or obese children	16 weeks of training	Significant increases in moderate-to-vigorous physical activity. Both groups exhibited significant reductions in percentage overweight and BMI, but the VG group exhibited significantly greater BMI reductions
O'Donovan et al. (2014)	Nintendo Wii	55 overweight or obese children	1 session	Certain VGs, particularly those that require lower limb movement, could be used to increase total energy expenditure, replace more sedentary activities, or achieve moderate intensity physical activity among children with obesity
Lau et al. (2015)	PlayStation 3 and Nintendo Wii	21 children	1 session	VG could provide alternative opportunities to enhance children's physical activity. They could be used as light-to-moderate physical activity, and with exergames, children can even reach the recommended intensity for developing and maintaining cardiorespiratory fitness

Table 4.7 Summary of studies about specific rehabilitation games included in this review on obesity and overweight

Study and Year	Subjects	Interventions	Outcomes
Jago et al. (2006)	473 boys (no weight criteria)	9 weeks of intervention though Internet for modifying food preferences and intake	No difference in body composition between groups
Doyle et al. (2008)	80 overweight or obese patients	16 weeks of Internet program for modifying food preferences and intake	BMI reduction after intervention but not 4 month after the intervention
Hung et al. (2008)	37 overweight patients	14 weeks of interventions program for modifying food preferences and intake	BMI, waist circumference, and triceps skinfold was reduced improve fitness, self-esteem, and self-efficacy
Jones et al. (2008)	105 subjects	16 weeks of Internet-based healthy weight maintenance program with mentor program	Reduction of BMI for intervention, binge eating behaviors, and weight and shape concerns but no change in dietary fat and sugar intake
Adamo et al. (2010)	30 overweight or obese adolescent	10 weeks, 2 sessions of 60 min a week of games, or a group of physical activity	No difference between group
Chen et al. (2011)	54 normal, overweight, or obese	Web-based information, diet, and physical activity	Decrease of waist and hip perimeter, modification of food intake
Christison and Khan (2012)	48 overweight or obese patients	10 weeks, 2 sessions of 60 min a week of games, or a group of physical activity	Significantly reduced television time and soda consumption while increased PA time and eating at the table. Significantly improved global self-worth and behavioral conduct
Wagener et al. (2012)	40 subjects	Supervised 10-weeks group dance-based exergame exercises or waitlist control group	No difference in pre-/post-test BMI improved self-perceived psychological adjustment and competence to exercise

between 1.5 and 2 kg after this intervention (Johnston et al. 2012). An important point of the rehabilitation, besides weight loss, is to change the behavior of patients and empower them in the self-management of their disease. The previous study also shows that patients are more active after the intervention, proof that they have realized the importance of performing physical activity in order to control their weights. This effect was also demonstrated in another study where games were introduced in physical education classes. The authors showed that 86 obese children who participated in this study were more active after this intervention (Quinn 2013).

Another interesting study was conducted to compare which kind of games, competitive games and cooperative games, was the most effective. 31 obese subjects

Fig. 4.6 Repartition of the devices for studies on obesity and overweight

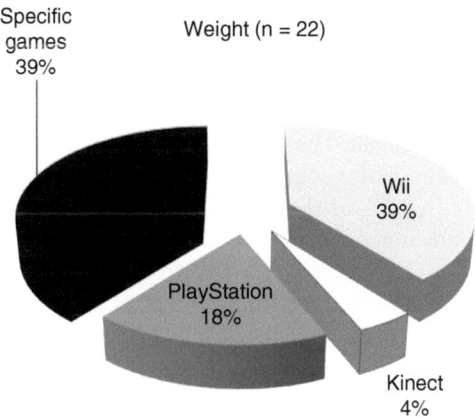

participated in this study. After 6 months of training (5 sessions per week), the authors found that patients who were playing games in cooperative mode had a higher intrinsic motivation and the level of intrinsic motivation was directly correlated with the level of energy expenditure (Staiano et al. 2012a, b). The same authors conducted another study with a control group. Patients in cooperative games group lost significantly more weight than both patients in the control group and those playing competitive games. Surprisingly, patients in the competitive group games did not lose weight (Staiano et al. 2013)!

It is also interesting to note that games can be used to help patients to control weight during temporary situations such as sports injuries, pregnancy, or postpartum (LeBlanc et al. 2013).

A study has been conducted on 34 women during the postpartum period. Subjects were divided into an intervention group and a control group. After 40 days of games, the authors observed a significant decrease in weight but also of the circumferences of the waist and thighs and the percentage of fat only in the intervention group. The authors also observed a significant decrease in calorie intake. The games could therefore lead to both an increase in energy expenditure and a decrease of energy intake. There is, naturally, a positive correlation between the amount of hours spent on the games and the weight loss. The authors concluded by stating that playing has fortunately (!) no influence on how the mother took care of their babies. (Tripette et al. 2014).

4.4 Stroke

4.4.1 Clinical Presentation

Stroke occurs when part of the brain is suddenly deprived of blood supply. This deficit causes a loss of function of the affected area of the brain. The severity of the disability and the degree of recovery depend on the extent, the localization of the lesions, and the time. Time is the key factor in the management of stroke. It is estimated that brain cells cannot survive for more than 3 min being deprived of oxygen without causing irreversible damage. Stroke is the third leading cause of death in the world and the leading cause of disability and long-term serious complications. It is estimated that 33 million of new cases of stroke are occurring each year (Samai and Martin-Schild 2015). Among the new cases about 10% of the patients will recover completely, 25% with mild deficits, 40% with moderate to severe deficits, 10% of these patients must be placed in specialized centers because of the functional impact, and 15% die shortly after stroke.

There are two types of strokes: ischemic and hemorrhagic.

Ischemic strokes are the most common (about 80% of cases); they are due to blood clots migration from peripheral artery to a clotted artery in the brain which will therefore become clogged when the diameter is too narrow. Most frequently, these clots are due to atherosclerosis: the accumulation of body fat (mainly cholesterol) in the arterial walls. This slowly causes loss of elasticity of the artery walls, a decrease in the light of the arteries (stenosis), and therefore blood flow reduction. This reduction may be up to the complete obliteration of the vessel (thrombosis) resulting in the death of the tissue located downstream of the thrombosis. Finally, the clot may crack and be released into the bloodstream.

The risk factors for ischemic stroke are age (75% of strokes occur after age 65), gender (incidence was 1.25 times higher for men), hypertension (80% of strokes occur in patients with hypertension [blood pressure greater than 140/90 mmHg]), diabetes (increasing the risk of a factor of 3.5 in women and 2.1 in men), hyperlipidemia and high cholesterol (HDL), smoking, sleep apnea, alcohol and drug use, and physical inactivity (low levels of physical activity) (Samai and Martin-Schild 2015).

Despite the fact that the majority of these risk factors are modifiable, and that awareness campaigns provide information on these risk factors, a significant increase in the new case of stroke is still observed (Stroebele et al. 2011). This increase is approximately 15% over the last 10 years.

Hemorrhagic strokes are due to a rupture of a cerebral artery. The major risk factor for hemorrhagic stroke is high blood pressure (Biffi et al. 2015).

4.4.2   Rehabilitation

Primary care, management, and rehabilitation after stroke are best examples of teamwork in physical rehabilitation. The first goal of rehabilitation is the autonomy.

Autonomy is defined as the right and/or the ability of a person to lead his life according to his free judgment. The second objective is to coordinate all measures to prevent or minimize the related functional potential consequences of the disease from a physical, psychological, social and economic point of view. The aim is to exploit and maximize the residual capacity of the patient. This approach differs from curative medicine by its multidisciplinary nature: the medical doctor has the role of coordinator of functional rehabilitation team, centered around participatory patient. The multidisciplinary rehabilitation team may consist of nurses, physio-therapists, occupational therapists, psychologists, speech therapists, social workers, dieticians, and neuropsychologists (Heuschling et al. 2013) (see Sect. 2.1.1).

Damages in the central nervous system causes spasticity in the limbs. Spasticity is an exaggeration of the tendon reflex activity. In case of voluntary contraction and motion, the muscle-tendon reflex activity is over exaggerated, muscles are too con-tracted, and therefore no more motion is possible.

During the rehabilitation, it is important to differentiate the acute phase (less than 3 months after the accident) and the chronic state. Treatment and recovery possibili-ties are indeed different.

In the acute phase, it is essential to start the rehabilitation process as soon as pos-sible to avoid adverse effect as much as possible that could affect the function and limit the disability. The first month after the stroke is a crucial period during which brain plasticity and thus recovery capabilities are maximized.

One of the main objectives of the stroke care unit is to minimize the impact of the induced spasticity from a functional point of view. Spasticity is also responsible for vicious postures because the muscles do not relax sufficiently. Reduction of the spasticity can be obtained with oral medication (e.g., Baclofen), by muscular injec-tion of Botulinum toxin, with intrathecal Baclofen (directly into the spinal canal), with casting or orthoses and physiotherapy. These approaches can, and should, be combined.

4.4.3 Use of Serious Games

Summary of the different studies included are presented in Tables 4.8 and 4.9 for commercial video games and specific ones, respectively. 53 studies were found in the literature. Repartitions of devices and approaches are presented in Fig. 4.7.

The most used systems are the Nintendo Wii and some specific solutions. Only three studies were performed using the PlayStation, including the first study in this area in 2008 (Yavuzer et al. 2008). Kinect was available only 5 years after the Nintendo Wii; therefore, there are fewer studies conducted with this device but there is a significant increase since 2013 and currently the recent studies are conducted with both devices equally.

During the acute rehabilitation, the use of games is justified by the need to per form as many repetitions of revalidation exercises as possible during the months following the stroke in order to maximize the chance of full recovery. We have already discussed the positive effects of games on motivation but it has also been shown that the games allow more repetitions of movement before patients get tired. Two studies were conducted to determine which devices allowed the highest repeti-tions of movements. The number of repetitions were compared using the PlayStation 3 and Wii with a group of stroke patients and a control group, a larger number of repetitions was observed for the PlayStation compared to the Wii and the intensity of the movements was also more important (Neil et al. 2013). Another study com-pared the number of movements using with the PlayStation 2, the Wii, and some

Table 4.8 Summary of studies about commercial video games included in this review on stroke rehabilitation

Study and Year	Device	Subjects	Interventions	Outcomes
Yavuzer et al. (2008)	PlayStation 2	20 patients with chronic stroke separated into intervention and conventional therapy group	4 weeks of training, 5 sessions per week	Significant improvement in the functional independent measure. No difference in Brunnstrom stages
Yong Joo et al. (2010)	Nintendo Wii	20 acute patients (less than 3-month post stroke)	2 weeks of training, 3 sessions per week	Statistically significant improvement in Fugl-Meyer assessment and Motricity index score
Saposnik et al. (2010)	Nintendo Wii	20 acute patients separated into intervention and conventional therapy group	2 weeks of training, 4 sessions per week	Significant improvement in mean motor function and stroke severity
Hurkmans et al. (2011)	Nintendo Wii	10 patients with chronic stroke	1 session	Patients playing Wii Sport experiment moderate intensity exercises
Mouawad et al. (2011)	Nintendo Wii	7 patients with chronic stroke and 5 healthy control	10 sessions during 10 consecutive days	Significant and clinically relevant improvement in functional motor ability
Cho et al. (2012)	Nintendo Wii	11 patients with chronic and 11 controls	6 weeks of training, 5 sessions per week	Significant improvement in dynamic balance for chronic patient, no difference in static balance
Celinder and Peoples (2012)	Nintendo Wii	9 patients	3 weeks of training, 1 to 9 sessions	Increase motivation and may benefit patient rehabilitation directly
Lee (2013a, b)	Xbox Kinect	14 acute patients (less than 6-month post stroke) separated into intervention and conventional therapy group	6 weeks of training, 3 sessions per week	Significant improvement in muscle strength of the upper extremities (except the wrist) and performance of activity of daily living
Kafri et al. (2013)	Nintendo Wii and Xbox Kinect	11 patients and 8 healthy controls	4 sessions of training over a week	Playing upper extremities or mobility VG resulted in moderate energy expenditure and intensity
Peters et al. (2013)	Nintendo Wii PlayStation 2	12 patients with chronic stroke	10 sessions of training	The number of repetitions is depending of the device (PlayStation > Nintendo Wii). Active gaming provided more upper extremity repetitions than for traditional therapy

Study	Device	Participants	Duration	Results
Neil et al. (2013)	PlayStation 3 Nintendo Wii	10 patients with chronic stroke and 10 healthy controls	1 session	The number of repetitions is depending of the device (PlayStation > Nintendo Wii). Greater movement intensity was found for the PlayStation 3 compared to Nintendo Wii
Rajaratnam et al. (2013)	Nintendo Wii Xbox Kinect	19 acute patients (less than 1-month post stroke)	3 weeks of training, 5 sessions per week	Improvement in functional mobility and balance
Sin et al. (2013)	Xbox Kinect	40 patients with chronic stroke separated into intervention and conventional therapy group	6 weeks of training, 3 sessions per week	Significant improvement in function of the upper limb
Bao et al. (2013)	Xbox Kinect	5 subacute patients	5 weeks of training, 3 sessions per week	Significant improvement in the Fugl-Meyer assessment and Wolf Motor Function
Barcala et al. (2013)	Nintendo Wii	20 patients with chronic stroke	5 weeks of training, 2 sessions per week	Significant improvement in body symmetry, balance, and function
Hung et al. (2014)	Nintendo Wii	30 patients with chronic stroke	12 weeks of training or conventional weight-shift training	The VG group shows more improvement in static balance than the control group. But the progresses were not maintained after 3 months. The exergaming group enjoyed training more than the control group
Choi et al. (2014)	Nintendo Wii	20 patients with subacute stroke	4 weeks of intervention (VG or occupational therapy), 5 sessions per week	No difference between group after intervention. These findings suggested that the commercial gaming-based VG therapy was as effective as conventional occupational therapy on the recovery of upper extremity motor and daily living function in subacute stroke patients
Subramaniam et al. (2014)	Nintendo Wii	8 community-dwelling individuals with hemiparetic stroke	VG training in conjunction with cognitive training, 110 min a day during 5 days	The results demonstrate good adherence and evidence of clinical value of this high-intensity, short-duration protocol for reducing cognitive-motor interference and improving balance control in stroke survivors

(continued)

Table 4.8 (continued)

Study and Year	Device	Subjects	Interventions	Outcomes
Morone et al. (2014)	Nintendo Wii	50 patient with stroke	4 weeks of balance training using VG or conventional balance therapy, 3 sessions per week	Wii Fit training was more effective than usual balance therapy in improving balance and independency in activity of daily living
Bower et al. (2014)	Nintendo Wii	30 patients with stroke	2 to 4 weeks of training for balance training (standing position) or upper limb rehabilitation (sitting position), 3 sessions per week	Wii use by the balance group was associated with trends for improved balance, with significantly greater improvement in outcomes including the step test and Wii balance board-derived center of pressure scores. The upper limb group had larger, nonsignificant changes in arm function
Shiner et al. (2014)	Nintendo Wii	10 patients with chronic stroke	14 days program of Wii-based upper limb rehabilitation with or without bilateral priming before the games	Bilateral priming before Wii-based movement therapy led to a greater magnitude and retention of improvement compared to control. Bilateral priming can enhance the efficacy of wii-based movement therapy
Viana et al. (2014)	Nintendo Wii	20 patients with chronic stroke	15 sessions of training using VG with or without transcranial direct current simulation	Both groups demonstrated gains in motor function. Wrist spasticity was significantly more decreased in the group with transcranial direct simulation
Fernandes et al. (2014)	Xbox Kinect	20 patients with stroke and 20 healthy subject	1 session	After the training, only patients with right brain injury improved their shoulder and elbow angles, approaching the left upper limb movement pattern of healthy subjects
Choi et al. (2014)	Nintendo Wii	20 chronic patients	4 weeks of training, 7 sessions per week	Significant improvement in Fugl-Meyer assessment, manual function test, box and block test, activities of daily living, cognitive function, and grip strength

Morone et al. (2014)	Nintendo Wii	50 subacute stroke patients	4 weeks of training, 3 sessions per week	Balance training with VG as a complement to conventional therapy was found to be more effective than conventional therapy alone in improving balance and reducing disability in patients with subacute stroke
Hung et al. (2014)	Nintendo Wii	30 chronic patients	12 weeks of training	Significant improvement in the timed up-and-go test, forward reach test, and fear of falling. The improvement in fear of falling was not maintained over time. The VG group enjoyed training more than the control group
Bower et al. (2014)	Nintendo Wii	30 acute patients	2–4 weeks of training, 3 sessions per week	Trends (not significant) towards improved balance and arm function
Lee et al. (2015)	Nintendo Wii	24 chronic patients	3 weeks of training, 3 sessions per week	Significantly more improvement in static balance and functional reach tests in the VG compared to control groups
Da Silva Ribeiro et al. (2015)	Nintendo Wii	30 chronic patients	3 weeks of training, 2 sessions per week	Significant improvement in Fugl-Meyer assessment and short-form health survey
Şimşek and Çekok (2016)	Nintendo Wii	42 acute patients	10 weeks of training, 3 sessions per week	Significant improvement in quality of life and daily living functions
Chen et al. (2015)	Nintendo Wii	24 chronic patients	8 weeks of training, 5 sessions per week	Significant improvement in Fugl-Meyer assessment. Patient enjoyment was significantly higher in the VG groups
Yatar and Yildirim (2015)	Nintendo Wii	30 chronic patients	4 weeks of training, 3 sessions per week	Significant improvement in balance, balance confidence, and activities of daily living
Omiyale et al. (2015)	Nintendo Wii	9 chronic patients	3 weeks of training, 3 sessions per week	Significant improvements in reaction time and balance confidence
Paquin et al. (2015)	Nintendo Wii	10 chronic patients	8 weeks of training, 2 sessions per week	Significant improvement in functional recovery, fine motor function, and quality of life
Song and Park (2015)	Xbox Kinect	40 chronic patients	8 weeks of training, 5 sessions per week	Significant improvement in balance, gait, and depression

Table 4.9 Summary of studies about specific rehabilitation games included in this review on stroke rehabilitation

Study and Year	Subjects	Interventions	Outcomes
Stewart et al. (2007)	2 chronic patients	12 training session over a 3 weeks period	Participants improved functional ability after training
Mirelman et al. (2010)	18 chronic patients	12 training session over a 3 weeks period	Subjects in the SG group demonstrated a significantly larger increase in ankle power generation at push-off as a result of training. The SG group had greater change in ankle ROM post-training as compared to the control group. Significant differences were found in knee ROM on the affected side during stance and swing, with greater change in the VR group
Ustinova et al. (2011)	13 patients with traumatic brain injury	1 session	Participants improved in game performance, arm movement time, and precision. Improvements were achieved mostly by adapting efficient arm-postural coordination strategies
Shiri et al. (2012)	6 acute patients	10 sessions of training	All participants succeeded in operating the system, demonstrating its feasibility in terms of adherence and improvement in task performance
Rabin et al. (2012)	5 chronic patients	6 weeks of training	Clinically significant improvements in their active range of shoulder movement, shoulder strength, grasp strength, and their ability to focus
Turolla et al. (2013)	376 chronic patients	20 sessions over a 4 weeks period	Both treatments significantly improved Fugl-Meyer upper extremity and functional independence measure scores, but the improvement obtained with VR rehabilitation was significantly greater than that achieved with conventional therapy
Orihuela-Espina et al. (2013)	8 chronic patients	/	Patients demonstrated significant behavioral improvements (Fugl-Meyer and Motricity index)
McEwen et al. (2014)	59 chronic patients	20 sessions over a 3 weeks period	Patients demonstrated significant improved mobility-related outcomes (timed up-and-go the two-minute walk test)

Study	Participants	Training	Results
Shin et al. (2014)	23 acute or subacute patients	10 sessions over a 2 weeks period	The SG intervention improved the Fugl-Meyer and the modified Barthel index
Lee and Chun (2014)	23 subacute patients	15 sessions over a 3 weeks period	The combination of brain stimulation and peripheral arm training using SG could facilitate a stronger beneficial effect on UE impairment than using each intervention alone
Cho et al. (2014)	10 chronic patients	2 weeks of training	Significant improvement in proprioception after the training
Tsekleves et al. (2014)	3 chronic patients	2 weeks of training	Participants reporting better wrist control and greater functional use
Kiper et al. (2014)	44 chronic patients	20 sessions over a 4 weeks period	The Fugl-Meyer and the functional independence measure scores were significantly higher in the SG group after treatment, but not speed-related parameters
Iosa et al. (2015)	4 subacute patients	6 sessions of 30 min	Patients showed a significantly higher improvement in hand abilities and grasp force
Bower et al. (2015)	40 chronic patients	4 weeks of training, 2 sessions per week	Acceptability was high for the intervention group and improvements over time were seen in several functional outcome measures. There were no serious adverse safety events reported
Joo et al. (2015)	38 subacute patients	5 weeks of training, 3 sessions per week	Significant short-term effects of the SG program on pulmonary function in stroke patients were recorded in this study
Shin et al. (2015)	35 chronic hemiparetic patients	4 weeks of training, 5 sessions per week	SG rehabilitation has specific effects on health-related quality of life, depression, and upper extremity function among patients with chronic hemiparetic stroke
Standen et al. (2015)	17 chronic patients	8 weeks of training, 3 sessions of 20 min per day	A weak positive correlation between duration and baseline reported activities of daily living. Participants reported lack of familiarity with technology and competing commitments as barriers to use although they appreciated the flexibility of the intervention and found it motivating

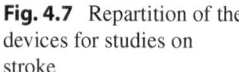

Fig. 4.7 Repartition of the devices for studies on stroke

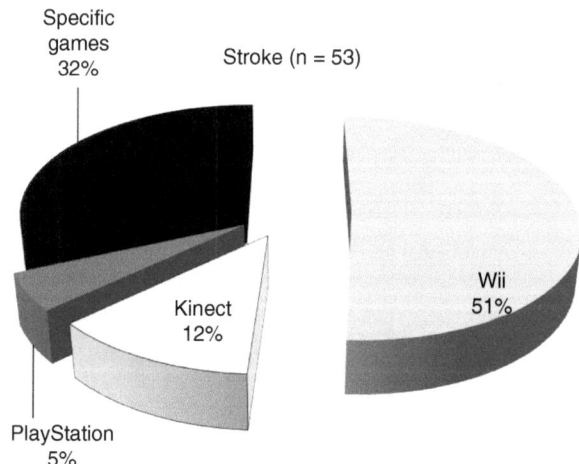

traditional rehabilitation exercises. The results are similar to those found in the previous study (PlayStation > Wii), but in both cases the active video games allow much more repetitions of movements than traditional exercises (Peters et al. 2013).

Another study quantified the difference in the amount of exercise performed with the Wii compared to traditional exercises. The movements were recorded during traditional rehabilitation session and during a session using video games. A physician determined whether the movements performed were voluntary or simple reflex movements. With the games the patients were performing an average of 271 movements against only 48 voluntary movements during traditional rehabilitation exercises. Therefore, patients perform nearly six times more exercise when playing games! If we keep in mind that the number exercises is one of the most important criteria in recovery after stroke (Langhorne et al. 2011), it is legitimate and appropriate to consider the fact of integrating these techniques in the rehabilitation of these patients. Patients with better prognosis performed more repetitions (Rand et al. 2014).

During the acute phase of the rehabilitation studies are generally performed over a period of 4 to 6 weeks after the stroke, the number of session varied between 3 and 5 times per week. Significant improvements are found for gross motor function (Saposnik et al. 2010, Yong Joo et al. 2010), balance (Rajaratnam et al. 2013), and muscle strength (Lee 2013a).

During the chronic phase, the interventions are usually longer. Positive effects were also found for static (Hung et al. 2014) and dynamic balance (Cho et al. 2012, Morone et al. 2014) and upper limb fine motor function (Sin and Lee 2013).

Concerning the development and use of specific solutions, many of these solutions involved robotic systems (haptic devices) or the development of treadmill combining virtual reality and games (immersion). These approaches are beyond the scope of this book and even if this is also a very interesting field of research and development we are not going to discuss and these studies here. Some notions on rehabilitation using haptic systems are presented in Sect. 7.3.

Mirror therapy is one of the techniques available for the rehabilitation of patients suffering from various neurological disorders, including stroke.

This technique is used in cases of asymmetric pathologies (e.g., amputation, hemiplegia, complex regional pain syndrome). The aim is to mislead the brain by reflecting the image of the healthy and movable limb onto the affected limb. The brain believes that the affected limb can move again and new connections could be created through visual stimuli. It could compensate the lack of sensory stimuli due to the disease or the absence of limb.

This technique could be easily applied using the virtual reality; the purpose is also to mislead the brain by creating virtually a false situation. Specific games have been developed: the patient moves the healthy limb and the game returns feedback indicating that the affected limb is mobilized and has influenced the game. Games have been developed and successfully tested for revalidation of the upper limbs based on mirror therapy (Shiri et al. 2012).

The developed solutions that offer an augmented visual feedback are based on the same principle: the aim is to prove to the brain that the body is still able to perform motions and exercises. Compared to conventional treatment, it has been observed that patients doing rehabilitation exercises using a system that provided enhanced feedback have a more favorable recovery of the upper limbs function (Kiper et al. 2014). Based on the same principle, it is possible to directly influence the brain (motor and sensory cortex) using transcranial stimulation during the use of revalidation exercises with serious games. A study was conducted on 59 patients during 3 weeks (5 sessions per week) to compare the use of video games coupled to transcranial stimulation, the use of video games alone, and one group receiving only transcranial stimulation. Although the three groups show improvement in various studied parameters, best results were obtained in the group receiving transcranial stimulation during the games (Lee and Chun 2014).

We already saw that the use of feedback or additional brain stimulus could have a positive clinical effect but using only games is also effective. Positive results were obtained in terms of mobility and balance after daily training (games focused on the lower limbs) during a 3 weeks period compared with conventional therapy, 59 patients participated in this study (McEwen et al. 2014). Concerning the upper limbs one study involving 376 patients had compared the effects of games coupled with the traditional rehabilitation compared to traditional rehabilitation exercises only. After 4 weeks of training (5 sessions per week), both groups show increases in mobility and independence but the results were significantly higher in the group that received games (Turolla et al. 2013).

A last point that needs to be addressed is to determine whether it is possible to predict what type of patient might mostly benefit from this type of intervention. Studies have been conducted using the functional magnetic resonance imaging (fMRI) to determine areas of the brain activated and the different strategies of neuronal reorganization after the stroke. After training with video games, it has been observed that the activities in the prefrontal cortex and in the cerebellum are the most predictive for motor recovery. One study on the relationship between movement and brain changes shows that the most disabled patients could obtain the most benefit from this new paradigm (Orihuela-Espina et al. 2013).

Another study performed with the Kinect during only one session shows that after this short training only patients that presented a lesion in the right hemisphere showed an increase of the mobility of shoulder and elbow and presented a pattern of motion closer than the healthy individuals (Fernandes et al. 2014).

The use of video games in stroke patients could therefore be used in clinic but more works are still needed to define the best protocols and better target patient (using functional imaging) and population that may benefit the most from these new intervention.

4.5   Balance Training

4.5.1   Clinical Presentation

Balance impairments are not diseases but a symptom found in many medical conditions. Proper balance control requires the integrity of three major systems: the vestibular system, the visual system, and the somatosensory system. The integration and synchronization of the different signals from these systems by the central nervous system must also be optimal.

The vestibular system is composed of the vestibule and the cochlea, located at the inner ear. Otoliths (cilia) and the semicircular canals inform the brain of the position of the head. Pathologies at this level (e.g., benign vertigo, neuroma of the eighth cranial nerve, vestibular neuritis) cause dizziness, loss of balance, nausea, and vomiting.

The visual system directly affects the balance by providing information about position of the body and movements. The information from the visual and vestibular systems are closely linked through the visual-vestibular integration. If there is a mismatch between the information from these two systems, dizziness occurs because the brain cannot interpret these conflicting signals and therefore cannot know the exact position of the head in space (i.e., driving a car on a mountain road).

Any disease that produces a loss of visual acuity can potentially lead to balance disorders (e.g., scotoma with the elderly).

The somatosensory system informs the brain about the forces applied on the body (touch, pressure, vibration) and the position of the body in space (3D). There are many receptors in the body either in the skin, muscles, tendons, or ligaments. Information goes in the somatosensory cortex (parietal lobe) through nerves and spinal cord. Numerous diseases can disrupt the proper functioning of these nerve pathways either in the brain (e.g., stroke), the nerves (e.g., multiple sclerosis), or peripherally in case of joint immobilization or due to a lack of movement (e.g., bedridden patient).

4.5.2 Rehabilitation

Medical doctors treat the underlying pathology, and the purpose of the rehabilitation is to restore or increase the proprioception and the performance of all the systems involved in balance and posture. The proprioception must be trained properly: trunk orientation in space eyes closed, corrections of posture in front of a mirror, improvement of postural tone, and strengthening of the muscles.

Another important concept in balance rehabilitation is the notion of feedback. Feedback is essential to train proprioception. Patients should indeed be aware of the changes of the position of the different body parts in space. This is exactly what is happening with the active video games since the patient must perform movements with his body to interact with the game. Therefore, patients receive direct feedback of movements which improves proprioception and cognitive function.

4.5.3 Use of Serious Games

We already discussed the issue and challenge of balance training with the elderly, stroke patients, and for Parkinson's disease patients and will discuss multiple sclerosis patient in the next chapter.

The issue of training, or retraining, balance can be divided into two categories: improving the balance after a disease that causes balance impairment (rehabilitation) or trying to increase performance (sport training).

Only studies including patients are presented here.

Summary of the different studies included are presented in Tables 4.10 and 4.11 for commercial video games and specific ones, respectively. 42 studies were found in the literature. Repartitions of devices and approaches are presented in Fig. 4.8.

One of the most obvious pathologies inducing balance disorders is malformation or lower limb amputations. The feasibility of integrating video games in the treatment of lower limb amputees has been tested. After a period of 4 weeks (4 sessions a week), balance improvement was observed. However, as with many other studies the long-term effects of this intervention was not assessed; therefore, we do not know if the benefits achieved are maintained sustainably over time (Andrysek et al. 2012).

Another study has been conducted with patients presenting various diseases in the lower limbs. The treatment lasted over a period of 4 weeks with 3 sessions per week. Patients were divided into an intervention group using video games and a control group with conventional therapy. After the program, progresses were similar in both groups, indicating that the games could be an option (Sims et al. 2013). Another study was done on a group athletes with lower limbs injuries. The intervention was longer (10 weeks with 2 sessions per week). Once again progresses

Table 4.10 Summary of studies about commercial video games included in this review on balance rehabilitation

Study Year	Device	Subjects	Interventions	Outcomes
Nitz et al. (2010)	Nintendo Wii	10 healthy women	10 weeks of training, 2 sessions per week	Significant improvement in balance and lower limb muscle strength but no significant change in touch, vibration, proprioception, cardiovascular endurance, mobility, weight change, activity level and well-being
Andrysek et al. (2012)	Nintendo Wii	6 children and adolescents with unilateral lower limb amputations and 10 healthy children	4 weeks of training, 4 sessions per week	Immediate improvement of balance after VG, long-term retention remains unclear
Meldrum et al. (2012)	Nintendo Wii	26 subjects with balance impairment	1 session	Participants enjoyed playing VG and 88% would like to use VG in future rehabilitation
Singh et al. (2012)	Nintendo Wii	36 dwelling women separated into intervention and conventional therapy group	6 weeks of training, 2 sessions a week	Both groups demonstrated improvement therefore gaming console could be used as a balance training tool
Salem et al. (2012)	Nintendo Wii	40 children with developmental delay	10 weeks of training, 2 sessions per week	Significant improvements in single leg stance test and grip strength
Andrysek et al. (2012)	Nintendo Wii	6 children with unilateral lower limb amputation, 10 healthy children	4 weeks of training, 4 sessions per week	Significant improvement in balance after VG, long-term retention remains unclear
Siriphorn and Chamonchant (2015)	Nintendo Wii	16 young adults	8 weeks of training, 2 sessions per week	Significant increase in balance and strength
Gioftsidou et al. (2013)	Nintendo Wii	40 healthy subjects separated into intervention and conventional therapy group	8 weeks of balance program with Nintendo Wii or with traditional training.	Both groups demonstrated improvement therefore gaming console could be used as a balance training tool

Study	Console	Participants	Protocol	Results
Sims et al. (2013)	Nintendo Wii	28 subjects with history of lower limb injuries	4 weeks of training, 3 sessions per week with Nintendo Wii or with traditional training.	Both groups demonstrated improvement therefore gaming console could be used as a balance training tool
Sparrer et al. (2013)	Nintendo Wii	71 patients with acute vestibular neuritis separated into intervention and conventional therapy group	Number of sessions depending of the patient	The early used of visual feedback for balance training accelerated the recovery after peripheral labyrinthine disorders
Nilsagård et al. (2013)	Nintendo Wii	84 patients with multiple sclerosis separated into intervention and conventional therapy group	6 weeks of training, 2 sessions per week	In comparison with no intervention, a program of supervised balance exercise using VG did not render statistically significant differences
Momberg et al. (2013)	Nintendo Wii	29 children with poor motor performance separated into intervention and conventional therapy group	6 weeks of training, 3 sessions per week	Both groups improved on all balance tests but higher improvement was found in the intervention group
Brichetto et al. (2013)	Nintendo Wii	36 patients with multiple sclerosis separated into intervention and conventional therapy group	4 weeks of training, 3 sessions per week	Statistically significant improvement in the interventional group
Vernadakis et al. (2013)	Xbox Kinect	63 injured young athletes separate into intervention, conventional therapy and control	10 weeks of training, 2 sessions per week	Both intervention and conventional therapy showed significant improvement compared to control group. Enjoyment was higher in the intervention group
Ortiz-Gutiérrez et al. (2013)	Xbox Kinect	50 patients with multiple sclerosis separated into intervention and conventional therapy group	10 weeks of training, 4 sessions per week or conventional therapy	Significant improvement in the intervention group for balance and Tinetti test
Prosperini et al. (2013)	Nintendo Wii	36 multiple sclerosis patients	12 weeks of training, 4 sessions per week	Significant improvement in motor performance and static balance

(continued)

Table 4.10 (continued)

Study Year	Device	Subjects	Interventions	Outcomes
Jelsma et al. (2014)	Nintendo Wii	28 children with developmental coordination disorder	6 weeks of training, 3 sessions per week	Significant improvement in motor performance and dynamic balance
Cuthbert et al. (2014)	Nintendo Wii	20 patients with traumatic brain injury	4 weeks of training, 4 sessions per week	Significant improvement in static and dynamic balance
Vernadakis et al. (2014)	Xbox Kinect	63 injured young athletes	10 weeks of training, 2 sessions per week	Significant improvement in dynamic and static balance
Cone et al. (2015)	Nintendo Wii	40 healthy young adults	6 weeks of training, 3 sessions per week	Significant improvement in balance and of proceeding multiple sources of sensory information
Naumann et al. (2015)	Nintendo Wii	37 healthy young adults	4 weeks of training, 3 sessions per week	Significant increases in performance on the trained games, but no transfer to performance on the untrained device and no changes in COP path length in quiet stance
Robinson et al. (2015)	Nintendo Wii	56 multiple sclerosis patients	4 weeks of training, 2 sessions per week	Significant improvements in bipedal postural sway and disability
Kim and Heo (2015)	Nintendo Wii	20 patients with ankle instability	4 weeks of training, 3 sessions per week	Significant improvement in static and dynamic balance
Wall et al. (2015)	Nintendo Wii	5 patients with incomplete spinal cord injury	7 weeks of training, 2 sessions per week	Significant changes in gait speed and functional reach. Survey reports suggested improvements in balance, endurance, and mobility in daily tasks at home
Pau et al. (2015)	Nintendo Wii	27 multiple sclerosis patients	5 weeks of training, 5 sessions per week	Significant improvement in postural control system performance
Su et al. (2015)	Xbox Kinect	43 healthy adults	6 weeks of training, 3 sessions per week	Significant improvement in dynamic and static balance

Table 4.11 Summary of studies about specific rehabilitation games included in this review on balance rehabilitation

Study and Year	Subjects	Interventions	Outcomes
Giansanti et al. (2009)	9 healthy subjects	1 session	Significant balance improvement after the virtual reality immersion
Alahakone et al. (2010)	6 patients with spinal-cord injury	1 session	Significant reduction in trunk tilt angles after virtual reality immersion
Janssen et al. (2010)	20 patients with severe bilateral vestibular losses	1 session	No significant change in total body sway after the training
Sztum et al. (2011)	30 community-dwelling older adults	8 weeks of training, 2 sessions per week	Greater improvement in dynamic standing balance control compared with the typical exercise program were observed
Nanhoe-Mahabier et al. (2012)	20 patients with PD	5 sessions	Significant balance improvement (reduction of CoP sway)
Sun and Lee (2013)	23 healthy subjects	1 session	It is possible to assess dynamic balance through the VG
Grewal et al. (2013)	29 patients with diabetic peripheral neuropathy	Number of sessions depending of the patient	Visual feedback generated from the games with motor learning may be effective in improving postural stability in patients
Schoene et al. (2013)	37 older adults	8 weeks of training, 2–3 sessions per week	Step pad training can be safely undertaken at home to improve physical and cognitive parameters of fall risk in older people without major cognitive and physical impairments
Franco et al. (2013)	20 community dwelling elder	1 session	Significant improvement of balance during the gait
Wüest et al. (2014)	16 community dwelling elder	36 sessions of training	Results indicate that the intervention improves gait- and balance-related physical performance measures in untrained subjects
Schwenk et al. (2014)	33 community dwelling elder with risk of falls	4 weeks of training, 2 sessions per week	Significant improvement in gait and balance after the intervention
Caudron et al. (2014)	17 patients with PD	1 session	Significant improvement of postural orientation and stability
Halická et al. (2014)	20 young healthy adults	1 session	Significant balance improvement (reduction of CoP sway)
Grewal et al. (2015)	39 diabetics patients	4 weeks of training, 2 sessions per week	Significant balance improvement after the intervention

(continued)

Table 4.11 (continued)

Study and Year	Subjects	Interventions	Outcomes
Ma et al. (2015)	30 subjects with reduced foot sensation	1 session	Significant gait improvement (mobility), strength, and balance after virtual reality immersion
Byl et al. (2015)	30 patients with PD and post-stroke	6 weeks of training, 2 sessions per week	Significant balance improvement (reduction of CoP sway)

Fig. 4.8 Repartition of the devices for studies on balance training

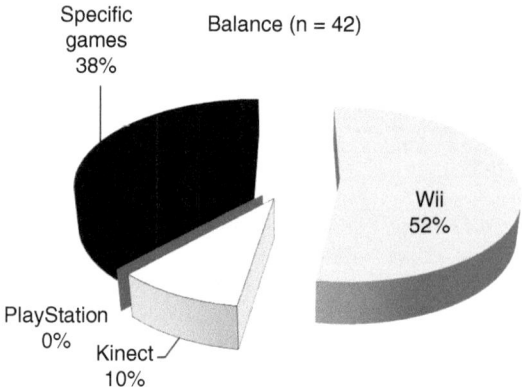

were similar in the video games group and in the group receiving standard treatment but the level of satisfaction was higher in patients who received the intervention with the games.

This type of intervention has also been tested in patients with acute vestibular neuritis. The duration of intervention was not similar for each patient but adapted according to the symptoms. Compared to conventional therapy, the authors observed that the early use of video games for the rehabilitation of the balance speeds up the process in case of peripheral lesion. These progresses would be due to the phenomenon of visual feedback provided by the games that has a positive effect on the visual-vestibular integration (Sparrer et al. 2013).

Meniere's disease is a pathology that also affects the inner ear (labyrinth). After 12 sessions of games and virtual reality, patients had less dizziness and an increase of the perimeter of stability and therefore a better quality of life (Garcia et al. 2013).

Patients with lower limb diseases could beneficiate from the use of video games. This might be due to the fact that patients prefer this kind of approach and are therefore performing more exercises since they are more fun.

In case of central pathologies of the inner ear, benefits and positive results are due to the neuronal plasticity and the increased integration of visual and vestibular information induced by visual feedback provided by the games.

4.6   **Cerebral Palsy**

4.6.1   **Clinical Presentation**

Cerebral palsy (CP) is a group of movement disorders that appears in the early childhood. CP is due to brain lesion occurring during pregnancy, childbirth, or during the first year of the children. These lesions, and therefore the movement disorders, are irreversible because these occurred on immature brain tissues. It is the leading cause of motor disability in pediatric. The prevalence is about 2 to 4 per 1000 living children (Winter et al. 2002). Patients suffering from CP present various motor and balance troubles. Depending on the type of underlying pathology (hemiplegia, diplegia, triplegia), upper and/or lower limbs can be affected. CP does not only lead to motor problem but also to sensitive issue (lack of proprioception, vision impairment, cognitive issue) that leads to difficulties in activities of daily living such as gait, posture, grasping, and fine motor control because of the underlying spasticity.

4.6.2   **Rehabilitation**

There is, currently, no specific treatment for CP patients. Research on stem cells and implantation of new cells in the nerve tissue slowly progresses in lab and research but are still far from being applied to patients. Management of children suffering from CP is a difficult and challenging task requiring various modifications throughout the revalidation process due to patients' evolution and growth.

The aim of the treatment is to increase the participation in activities of daily living, increasing the autonomy and decreasing the related side effect of the pathology such as bones deformations and muscles co-contraction that would lead to vicious posture.

The therapeutic approach and management of the spasticity related to CP is relatively similar to those used with stroke patient.

Adolescence is typically a difficult period for the rehabilitation of these patients. Indeed, they are already following heavy rehabilitation program since more than 10 years and some of them can question the benefits of this program. CP is an irreversible disease, therefore, the progresses—if any(!)—are really slow despite the important effort. During adolescence, patients do not want to do the exercises anymore because they think it is useless since they are not feeling any improvement. However, it is important to maintain a sufficient level of activity in order to maintain the benefits acquired during childhood but also in order to avoid decrease of general condition and bad or vicious attitudes induced by the spasticity.

The use of serious games during this difficult period could be particularly beneficial to struggle against this lack of motivation and the related negative consequences.

Another interesting period to introduce the games is the intensive rehabilitation period that follows a surgery or a Botox injection. After such kind of intervention, an intensive rehabilitation program of about 6 weeks is usually prescribed in order to maximize the benefits induced by the decrease of spasticity and to increase the range of motion and functions. Games offer an interesting alternative and motivational tool during this period.

4.6.3 Use of Serious Games

Summary of the different studies included are presented in Tables 4.12 and 4.13 for commercial video games and specific ones, respectively. 31 studies were found in the literature. Repartitions of devices and approaches are presented in Fig. 4.9. More than half of the studies are done using specially developed solutions for rehabilitation. This is due to the specific needs of the patients, the wide variety of symptoms, and due to functional abilities of these patients. Each patient is unique and therefore requires tailored rehabilitation programs.

First, let's discuss about the use of commercial video games.

The use of Xbox coupled with the Kinect has been integrated into conventional treatment over a period of 8 weeks with CP patients. After this period, improvement of motor functions (walking and balance) and fine motor skills has been observed. However, it is difficult to determine if the improvements are due to the specific effect of the games in revalidation or if it is simply due to the fact that the amount of rehabilitation has been increased by the integration of these exercises in the conventional treatment (Luna-Oliva et al. 2013).

More studies are available on the use of the Nintendo Wii and Balance Board. One study compared the integration of games (Nintendo Wii Sports) in the treatment; results were compared with conventional care. After this treatment, the patients had a significant improvement in the balance. Moreover, participation levels, satisfaction, and cooperation were also higher in the group receiving the intervention with the games compared to the control group (Sharan et al. 2012). The benefits of the games on the motivation and participation of CP children are clear and have been highlighted in various studies. On the other hands from a clinical point of view all the published studies using the Nintendo Wii did not find positive results. For example, a study has tested the integration of SG after surgery during 5 weeks (5 sessions of 30 min per week); no difference was found in terms of posture and balance before or after the intervention (Ramstrand and Lygnegård 2012). However, another study, performed over a period of 3 weeks (3 sessions per week), in which the games were used instead of physiotherapy, shows positive effects on the balance after this relatively short training period (Jelsma et al. 2013). To our knowledge, only one study was performed using the Wii controller instead of the Balance Board. The authors wanted to determine whether this kind of exercise could enhance upper limbs function. After a 12 weeks program (2 sessions per week), the authors did not find qualitative increase in upper extremity skills but they observed a significant increase in the use of the upper limbs for functional activities of daily living (Winkels et al. 2013).

Table 4.12 Summary of studies about commercial video games included in this review on cerebral palsy rehabilitation

Study and Year	Device	Subjects	Interventions	Outcomes
Jannink et al. (2008)	PlayStation 2	12 CP children	6 weeks of training	Children were happy to play VG but no difference was found with functional measurement
Hurkmans et al. (2010)	Nintendo Wii	8 adults with CP	1 session	The VG promote moderate intensity exercises
Sandlund et al. (2011)	PlayStation 2	15 CP children	4 weeks of training, daily training	The VG promote physical activity and enhance motor performance
Gordon et al. (2012)	Nintendo Wii	7 CP children	6 weeks of training, 2 sessions per week	Improvement in gross motor function measure
De Kloet et al. (2012)	Nintendo Wii	50 patients (child and young adults [6–29 years old]) with acquired brain injury	12 weeks of training, 2 sessions per week	Significant changes in physical activity, speed, and information processing. No difference in quality of life
Sharan et al. (2012)	Nintendo Wii	16 CP children after surgery	3 weeks of training	Significant improvement for balance. Participation, satisfaction, and cooperation were significantly higher in the VG group
Ramstrand et al. (2012)	Nintendo Wii	18 CP children	5 weeks of training for a minimum of 30 min a day 5 days a week	No significant difference was found for balance evaluation
Sandlund et al. (2012)	PlayStation 2	15 CP children	4 weeks of training, daily	Parent's perception about the use of VG for training was very positive
Luna-Oliva et al. (2013)	Xbox Kinect	11 CP children	8 weeks of training added to conventional physiotherapy treatment	Significant improvement in motor skills and fine dexterity
Robert et al. (2013)	Nintendo Wii	10 CP children and 10 control children	1 session of 40 min playing 4 different VG	The exercise intensity (heart rate) was similar for CP children and control

(continued)

Table 4.12 (continued)

Study and Year	Device	Subjects	Interventions	Outcomes
Jelsma et al. (2013)	Nintendo Wii	14 CP children	3 weeks of training instead of the conventional therapy	Significant improvement in balances score. Most of the children prefer VG compared to conventional treatment
Tarakci et al. (2013)	Nintendo Wii	14 CP children	12 weeks of training, 2 sessions per week	Statistically significant improvement in balance
Sandlund et al. (2014)	PlayStation 2	15 CP children	4 weeks of training for at least 20 min a day	Significant improvement in movement precision. Training with motion interactive games seems to improve arm motor control in children with CP
Chiu et al. (2014)	Nintendo Wii	62 CP children	6 weeks of training	No difference in coordination and hand function after the intervention
Al Saif and Alsenany (2015)	Nintendo Wii	40 CP children	12 weeks of training, 7 sessions per week	Significant improvement in motor performance compared to a control group
Zoccolillo et al. (2015)	Xbox Kinect	22 CP children	4 weeks of training, 4 sessions per week	Significant improvement in upper limb motor function but no improvement in fine motor function during activities of daily living

Finally, the PlayStation has also been tested. The first study was conducted to determine if the games could be used to promote physical activity and gross motor control. After a period of 4 weeks (5 sessions per week), an increase of motor performance was observed. The intensity level reached during the games corresponds to a mild to moderate physical activity (Sandlund et al. 2011). The same team repeated this protocol focusing on the precision of movements and fine motor skills (upper limbs). They observed an improvement in the precision and fluidity of movements during the game (Sandlund et al. 2014). Unfortunately, the authors did not evaluate whether the progress observed in the game was transferred to activity of daily living.

The specifically developed applications are mainly focused on the rehabilitation of the upper limbs. Unfortunately, the majority of these studies are performed with a very small number of children (3–4); therefore, it is difficult to determine if such

Table 4.13 Summary of studies about specific rehabilitation games included in this review on cerebral palsy rehabilitation

Study and Year	Subjects	Interventions	Outcomes
Akhutina et al. (2003)	66 CP children (7–14 years old)	6 to 8 sessions of 30–60 min during one month in the intervention group. Nonspecific rehabilitation training in the control group	No difference was observed between groups in the computer based tests. More important improvement in the intervention group for Benton judgment of line orientation test, arrows subtest of the Nepsy, roads test compared to control group
Reid (2005)	13 CP children (8–13 years old)	8 sessions of 60 min of SG play intervention	SG environment stimulated playfulness of CP children
Harris and Reid (2005)	16 CP children (8–12 years old)	8 sessions of 90 min of SG play interventions	SG seems to be a promising medium for the delivery of a motivating rehabilitation program
Reid and Campbell (2006)	31 CP children (8–10 years old)	One session of 90 min of SG per week during 8 weeks (soccer, volleyball, music). Standard care in the control group	No statistically significant difference was found except for the social acceptance (subscale of the self-perception profile) for children showing a significant improvement in SG intervention group
Chen et al. (2007)	4 CP children (6.3 years old)	4 weeks intervention program (2 or 3 session per week for a total of 120 min of treatment per week) added to regular therapies programs. The SG was focused on hand rehabilitation training system	3 of the 4 children showed improvement in the quality of reaching performance, training effect were partially maintained 4 weeks after the intervention. Increase in the fine motor domain
Golomb et al. (2010)	3 children with hemiplegic CP (13–15 years old)	Minimum 30 min of SG a day five days a week during 3 months	Improvement in function of the plegic hand and in bones' density. fMRI show spatial extent of activation relative to baseline in brain motor circuitry
Kirshner et al. (2011)	16 CP children (9 ± 2 years old) and a control group of 16 typically developing children (9 ± 2 years old)	Two 60 min sessions in 2 weeks, 4 different games were tested	Both groups enjoyed playing the games (no difference between groups). CP children have lower score (performance) during the games

(continued)

Table 4.13 (continued)

Study and Year	Subjects	Interventions	Outcomes
Wu et al. (2011)	12 CP children (8 years old)	18 sessions of 60 min training (20 min of warm-up and passive stretching, 15 min of assisted-active movement, 15 min of resisted-active movement, 110 min of cool down passive-stretching)	Increase in AROM and PROM. Improvement in joint biomechanical properties, motor control performance, and functional capability in balance and mobility
Chen et al. (2012a, b)	28 children with hemiplegic CP (6–12 years old)	40 min of training (the program consisted of a 5 min warm-up exercise, twenty repetitions of sitting-to-standing movements, cycling for 20 min, and a cool-down exercise for 5 min.) a day 3 times per week for 12 weeks. General physical activity in the control group	Significant and large effect on knee muscle strength after the treatment compared to control. Both groups did not significantly differ in BOTMP and gross motor function after intervention
Ritterband-Rosenbaum et al. (2012)	40 children with hemiplegic CP (12 years old) and a healthy age-matched group of 65 children	30 min daily training using an Internet-based home training system for CP children (MiTii, MiTii development). General physical activity in the control group	Significantly larger increase in the number of correct subjective reporting and a decrease of compensatory motions in the reaching tasks
Green and Wilson (2012)	8 children with hemiparetic upper limb motor disorders (from 4 to 15 years old).	30 min of daily training using RE-ACTION system during 3 or 4 weeks.	Improvement of upper limb function and activity participation after rehabilitation
Chen et al. (2013)	27 CP children (age 6–12 years old)	40 min of cycling on a virtual cycling system, three times a week during 12 weeks. General physical activity in the control group.	CP in the intervention group had greater femoral bone mineral density and isokinetics torques of knee muscles. Muscle strengthening program coupled to virtual reality is more specific than general activity
Jaume-i-Capó et al. (2014)	9 adults with CP	20 min of balance training, once a week during 24 weeks	Significant increases in balance and gait function scores were found after the intervention. These results indicate a greater independence for the participants

Table 4.13 (continued)

De Mello Monteiro et al. (2014)	32 adults with CP (19 years old) and 32 healthy subjects in the control group	1 session in a virtual environment	The individuals with CP did—as did their typically developing peers—improve coincidence timing with practice on both tasks. Importantly, however, these improvements were specific to the practice environment; there was no transfer of learning
Bonnechère et al. (2015)	10 CP children	4 weeks of training, 1 session of 30 min integrated in the conventional treatment per week	Significant balance improvement (static and dynamic) after the intervention

Fig. 4.9 Repartition of the devices for studies on CP

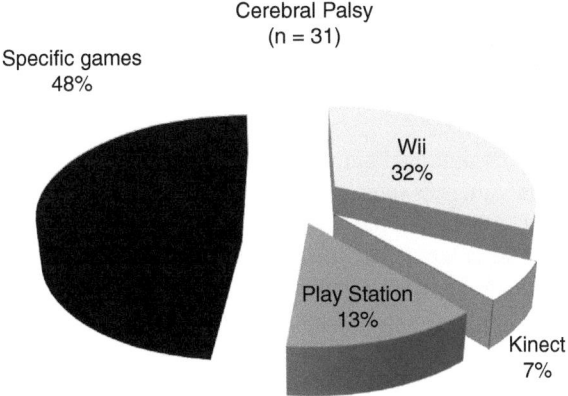

Cerebral Palsy
(n = 31)

Specific games
48%

Wii
32%

Play Station
13%

Kinect
7%

kind of solution can be used. Nevertheless, some feasibility studies show promising results. A study of 3 weeks (5 sessions per week) has been done with 3 children suffering from CP. The games were developed for the rehabilitation of the upper limbs and fingers (fine motor control). A significant increase in function of the affected limb and an increase in bone density was observed. Brain MRI shows an increase in the activation of the cerebral cortex after this training program (Golomb et al. 2010).

Another study was conducted with 8 patients for a 4 weeks training period (5 times a week). After the intervention, the authors observed a significant improvement in scores during the games but most interestingly they observed a transfer of the progresses in the games into upper extremity function and participation in activity of daily living (Green and Wilson 2012).

Considering the complexity of the disease, its management, and particularly negative impact of the loss of motivation during the conventional rehabilitation, the integration of games can be an interesting tool to encourage these children to perform the exercises. It has also been demonstrated that the games can stimulate neural brain circuits and could therefore allow additional benefits.

4.7   Parkinson's Disease

4.7.1   Clinical Presentation

Parkinson's disease is a neurodegenerative disease. The affected cells are located in the substantia nigra (the basal ganglia) of the brain (Fig. 2.1). The basal ganglia are involved in complex mechanisms of activation/inhibition in order to control the movements. The classical triad of symptoms is: rest tremor (tremor decreases when patients perform movements), increased rigidity, and akinesia (difficulty to initiate movements). Patients become gradually unable to perform movements accurately because of the increased stiffness and the progressive loss of control and coordination. The gait of patients suffering from Parkinson's disease is typical: first a flat foot strikes then progressively toe to heel walking. Balance and posture are also affected. Therefore, the risk of falls is increased.

Another factor that increases the risk of falling and limits patient's autonomy is the freezing. Freezing is the difficulty for patients to initiate movement or to continue rhythmic repetitive motions.

The prevalence of the disease increases with age. It is estimated that before 50 years it affects less than 2‰ of the population, 8‰ around 65, and about 35‰ after 85 years.

The aim of the treatment is to decrease the symptoms and the related negative consequences (e.g., loss of autonomy) since no substance is available yet to stop the degeneration of nerve cells.

Keystone of the oral medication is L-Dopa, a precursor of dopamine, normally produced in the substantia nigra.

4.7.2   Rehabilitation

Physiotherapists focus on the main symptoms of the disease: mainly the rigidity and the akinesia. The aim is to avoid associated complications: risk of falling, decreased independence, autonomy, and quality of life.

The aim is to preserve the function as much as possible and thus maintain the physical condition of patients to fight against inactivity. Being more active gives more confidence to patients and decreases the risk of falling. When the pathology is more advanced (when freezing occurs), more attention is paid to cognitive strategies. The use of feedback can be used to fight against akinesia and promote the initiation of movements. These different situations could be recreated in video games. Therefore, the games could provide interesting solutions for balance exercises as well as provide visual feedback to the patient.

4.7.3   Use of Serious Games

Summary of the different studies included are presented in Tables 4.14 and 4.15 for commercial video games and specific ones, respectively. 13 studies were found in the literature. Repartitions of devices and approaches are presented in Fig. 4.10.

Table 4.14 Summary of studies about commercial video games included in this review on Parkinson's disease

Study and Year	Device	Subjects	Interventions	Outcomes
Pompeu et al. (2012)	Nintendo Wii	32 PD patients	7 weeks of training, 2 sessions per week	Significant improvement in motor performance
Esculier et al. (2012)	Nintendo Wii	10 PD patients	6 weeks of training, 2 sessions per week	Significant improvement in static and dynamic balance, mobility, and functional abilities
dos Santos Mendes et al. (2012)	Nintendo Wii	16 early stage PD patients	14 weeks of training, 2 sessions per week	PD patients were able to transfer motor ability trained with VG to similar untrained tasks
Herz et al. (2013)	Nintendo Wii	20 PD patients	4 weeks of training, 3 sessions per week	Significant improvement in motor function, quality of life, and activities of daily living. Results were maintained months after playing VG
Gonçalves (2013)	Nintendo Wii	15 PD patients	7 weeks of training, 2 sessions per week	Significant increase in stride length and gait speed, reduction in motor impairments, and greater functional independence
Mhatre et al. (2013)	Nintendo Wii	10 PD patients	8 weeks of training, 3 sessions per week	Significant improvement in balance and gait, but no significant changes in activities specific to balance confidence or depression
Zalecki et al. (2013)	Nintendo Wii	24 PD patients	6 weeks of training, 2 sessions per week	Significant improvement in Berg Balance Scale, Tinnet's performance-oriented mobility assessment, timed up-and-go, sit-to-stand test, 10-meter walk test and activities-specific balance confidence scale
Pompeu et al. (2014)	Xbox Kinect	7 PD patients	5 weeks of training, 3 sessions per week	Significant improvement in activities (balance and gait), body functions (cardiopulmonary aptitude), and participation (quality of life)
Liao et al. (2015)	Nintendo Wii	36 PD patients	6 weeks of training, 2 sessions per week	Significant improvement in obstacle crossing performance and dynamic balance

Most of the studies have been conducted with the Nintendo Wii coupled with the Balance Board. Specific solutions have been gradually developed since 2013 and represent now about a quarter of the studies published in the field.

Parkinson's disease induces abnormal movement, especially the initiation of the motion, and balance disorders. The integration of games using the Wii in the rehabilitation program has a positive effect on both static and dynamic balance,

Table 4.15 Summary of studies about specific rehabilitation games included in this review on Parkinson's disease

Study and Year	Subjects	Interventions	Outcomes
Dowling et al. (2013)	20 PD patients	1 session	A computer-based video game that incorporates therapeutic movements to improve gait and balance for people with PD was appealing to subjects and feasible for home use
Van den Heuvel et al. (2014)	32 PD patients	5 weeks of training, 2 sessions per week	SG is a feasible and safe approach for balance rehabilitation but results are not superior over conventional balance training
Galna et al. (2014)	9 PD patients	1 session	It is safe and feasible for people with PD to use SG intervention to improve the postural control
Palacios-Navarro et al. (2015)	7 PD patients	5 weeks of training, 4 sessions per week	Significant improvements in completion of time score and the 10 meters walk test score

Fig. 4.10 Repartition of the devices for studies on Parkinson's disease

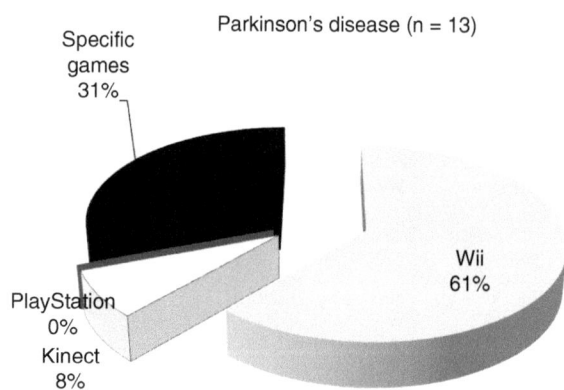

mobility, and function (Esculier et al. 2012, 2014, Pompeu et al. 2012). We already discussed the concept of specificity of rehabilitation exercises and the notion of transfer between these exercises and activities of daily living. A nice study showed that after 14 weeks of training (2 sessions per week), the patients were able to transfer the progresses they made during the games into relatively similar tasks of activity of daily living that had not been specifically trained during the rehabilitation using the games (dos Santos Mendes et al. 2012). Another important aspect of rehabilitation programs is to determine whether or not the progresses are acquired over a long period of time or just during the training period. One study showed that after a relatively short program (4 weeks, 3 sessions per week), patients had a significant increase in motor function during activities of daily living and augmented quality of life, these progresses were maintained 4 weeks (period equal to the duration of the intervention) after the rehabilitation program (Herz et al. 2013). Besides having an immediate impact on the balance and function, integrating games into the rehabilitation program seems therefore to induce long-term benefits.

The games have also a positive effect on the gait. After 7 weeks of training (2 sessions per week), there is an increase of stride length and walking speed and thus increased functional independence (Gonçalves 2013).

Using the Xbox Kinect was also tested first to ensure the feasibility and safety of this intervention with PD patients (Galna et al. 2014) then in a longer study (5 weeks 3 sessions per week) to evaluate the potential clinical effects. The games improve balance and walking, cardiopulmonary function as well as the quality of life (Pompeu et al. 2014).

Concerning the specific solutions, most of them are focusing on the rhythmicity of movements (Robles-Garcia et al. 2013) and the dual-task training (Su et al. 2015), two important kinds of rehabilitation exercises for PD patients. Solutions integrating virtual reality and visual feedback have also been developed. The aim is to provide an increased visual feedback to facilitate the integration of visual information in the vestibular-visual control loops (see Sect. 2.1.3). However, currently this kind of approach has not demonstrated superior efficacy compared to conventional rehabilitation program for balance with this kind of patients (van den Heuvel et al. 2014).

4.8 Orthopedic

After any type of orthopedic intervention (surgery, cast immobilization), rehabilitation sessions are prescribed. The aim of these sessions is to restore normal mobility and optimal joint functioning. After a surgery or immobilization muscles are atrophied, the joints are stiff and the proprioception is decreased. To avoid further complications, it is essential to restore these functions.

Currently, the development of serious games in the orthopedic field is mainly done in two pathologies: the management of low back pain and rehabilitation after prosthesis (hip and knee).

4.8.1 Low Back Pain

Low back pain can be acute (pain that lasts for less than 4 weeks), subacute (pain that lasts between 4 weeks and 3 months), or chronic (pain lasting for more than 3 months). Low back pain management depends on the type of pain and of the underlying pathology. It has been clearly demonstrated that, once again, the best approach is a multidisciplinary management of these patients. Many centers offer back schools program in which patients receive physiotherapy treatment, aerobic training (treadmill, bike, rowing machine), occupational therapy advices, and drug intervention, if the pain cannot be managed, as well as a psychological intervention.

Low back pain not only affects the patients physically, but also the quality of life (job loss, reduced social contact, poor sleep quality).

One of the objectives of the back school program is to teach the patient how to manage the pain in order to be more independent (patient empowerment). In the case of low back pain, perhaps more than in any other condition, it is essential that patients regularly perform home exercises to maintain the benefits achieved during the revalidation. Despite this need, only a few patients regularly perform such kind of exercises. It is indeed estimated that only 30% of patients actually perform the exercises prescribed by therapists (van Gool et al. 2005)!

Currently, the use of games is tested to try to increase compliance and adherence of patients to the prescribed exercises. In the future, the games will probably also be used to ensure that patients perform the exercise properly and be sure that they are doing it correctly (see Sects. 7.3.1 and 7.3.2).

The first study was conducted in 2013: a group of 24 low back pain patients were divided into three groups: a group with video games, a group with lumbar spine stabilization exercises, and a group receiving conventional treatment. After 8 weeks of intervention (3 sessions per week), the authors observed a significant increase in all the physical parameters (strength, walking distance) but also psychological (depression scale, sleep quality) in the first group while in two other groups improvements in physical parameters only were observed (Park et al. 2013). This study suggests that the use of games could have a beneficial effect on the related disorders associated with chronic low back pain.

Another study showed similar results after a 4 weeks training (also 3 sessions per week). 30 patients participated in this study and were separated into a group receiving treatment with the games and a group receiving conventional treatment. After the intervention, patients in the video game group had lower levels of pain than the conventional group and were also less afraid to move and perform physical activities (Kim et al. 2014).

4.8.2   Prosthesis

Some problems of an aging population (increased risk of falls, decreased cognitive functions, loss of strength and proprioception) have already been addressed. Osteoarthritis (progressive deterioration of articular cartilage that leads to pain and a decrease of the walking distance and autonomy) can be added to this list. The most commonly affected joints are the hip and knee. Once the joint is too damaged the treatment is prosthesis (total or partial depending on the severity). To prevent muscle atrophy and stiffness of the joints, mobilization must occur as soon as possible after the surgery. In case of total knee prosthesis, mobilizations already took place the first day after the intervention. For the hip prosthesis, it takes two or three days before performing weight-supported exercises.

We already discussed the positive effect of exercise training on psychological functions with low back pain patients (Park et al. 2013). It would also be possible to achieve changes in physical function by doing mental training. One study has indeed highlighted the positive effect of a daily 12 days mental training program with the game "How old is your brain" directly after total hip replacement.

After this program, patients in the intervention group presented more favorable clinical evolution compared to the control group (Lehrl et al. 2012).

Performing mental activity improves the physical rehabilitation of patients after total hip replacement. This underlines the importance of neural plasticity and the complexity of the different neural circuits involved in the motor control.

Another study explores the feasibility and safety of incorporating active video games in revalidation after placement of total knee prosthesis. Fifty patients participated in this study. Fifteen minutes of video games were included in the conventional session (30 min) of physical therapy while the control group received 30 min of physical therapy. The authors did not reveal any significant difference between the groups for pain or function. The patients were equally satisfied with either procedure (Fung et al. 2012).

Finally, although it is not a study about the rehabilitation after prosthesis, it is worth mentioning this study about rehabilitation after reconstruction of the cruciate ligaments of the knee since it is also a very common surgery in orthopedics. 30 patients were included in this study and were divided into two groups: one receiving rehabilitation using video games and the other group receiving conventional treatment. After 12 weeks of revalidation (3 sessions per week), there was no difference between the two groups in terms of muscle strength, dynamic balance, and range of motion of the knee (Baltaci et al. 2013).

These two studies show that games could be integrated safely into treatment and in some cases even replace conventional treatment. Some patients obtained similar results with the games than with conventional care.

4.9   Other Pathologies

In this part, we will discuss various pathologies to show the wide range of different possible interventions. The list of these pathologies is obviously not exhaustive.

4.9.1   Multiple Sclerosis

Multiple sclerosis, MS, is a disease affecting the central nervous system. This is an autoimmune disease that affects the myelin sheath surrounding the nerves. Myelin serves to protect the nerves but also and especially to increase the speed of propagation of nerve impulses.

Due to the high prevalence of the disease in the population, about 1/1000, this pathology could have been discussed in a chapter as well as for stroke or cerebral palsy but due to the limited number of studies in the domain we discuss it here.

The disease progresses as relapsing-remitting. Contrary to what have been thought for a long time, physical activity does not increase the risk of triggering a relapse. It is therefore recommended to increase the physical activity level of the patient. The level of activity must be adapted to the patients' abilities because it has been shown that the decline of the disease was slower when the physical activity level was higher.

Before discussing the clinical efficacy, a team of researchers studied the impact of the use of games on self-confidence and in quality of life. After 40 sessions of training, they observed that patients that are using the games had more confidence in their ability to achieve physical goals and to participate in recreational activities. The games allow the patient to train without having to go to a physiotherapist or a gym. The study also highlights the fact that one must be careful during the first sessions with the games because patients are intimidated by playing games and are afraid of falling (Gutiérrez et al. 2013).

Regarding the clinical efficacy, two studies have been identified with the Wii Balance Board. The first did not show any positive effect of training (12 sessions over 6 weeks) compared with a group of patients that did not perform exercises (Nilsagård et al. 2013). By cons in the second study, also after a 12 sessions training (4 weeks), the authors demonstrate a significant increase in the balance after the intervention compared to a group following a conventional rehabilitation (Brichetto et al. 2013).

The same positive results on balance were found after training 40 sessions (10 weeks) conducted with the Xbox Kinect compared with conventional treatment (Ortiz- Gutiérrez et al. 2013).

4.9.2 Fibromyalgia

Fibromyalgia is defined by widespread pain throughout the whole body, general fatigue, and sleep disturbances (poor and non-restorative sleep). The origin of this disease is still not fully understood, and the therapeutic management remains controversial. Besides drug therapy (e.g., pain, depression), it is important for the patients to stay active despite the fact that exercise could exacerbate the pain. Some studies have been conducted on the use of serious games in the treatment of this pathology.

Six women with fibromyalgia participated in this study. After 10 sessions, the researchers observed a significant decrease in pain and depression. It is interesting to note that these positive results were maintained 6 months after the intervention (Botella et al. 2013).

Another study was conducted on the potential psychological effects of the games: quality of life, emotions, coping strategies (in psychology, it is an individual's strategy for dealing with stress). The purpose of this study was to promote positive emotions and coping strategies. The results show a significant increase in general health, positive emotions, motivation, and self-esteem indicating that virtual reality can be used in the field of psychological care of patients with fibromyalgia (Herrero et al. 2014).

Finally, a study shows that, after 15 sessions of treatment, serious games can be integrated into the treatment of rehabilitation and have a positive effect on temporary pain reduction (Mortensen et al. 2015).

These studies show that the serious games could provide help in the treatment of fibromyalgia.

4.9.3   Systemic Lupus Erythematosus

Systemic lupus erythematosus is a systemic autoimmune disease (affecting the whole body). The connective tissue (supportive tissue that surrounds and protects the organs) are affected. Physiotherapy is important to fight against the related phenomena of arthritis (inflammation of the joints), joint pain, and tendinitis. Physical activity should also be encouraged to prevent global fatigue.

It affects mostly women (9 women for 1 men).

A group of researchers integrated the commercial video games (Wii Fit) in the conventional treatment of these patients. After an intervention of 10 weeks (3 sessions per week), they found a significant decrease in fatigue, weight, waist circumference, level of anxiety, and pain (Yuen et al. 2011). The same team continued the experiments and showed that games increased the motivation of patients and therefore adherence to treatment (Yuen et al. 2013).

4.9.4   Schizophrenia

Schizophrenia is a mental illness characterized by a loss of contact with reality related to some defects in neural circuits of the brain. There are many related disorders: attention, memory, concentration, deficits in executive functions (performing daily living activities). These disorders progressively induce difficulties in social life and activities for these patients. The management should include activities allowing the patient to take care of itself and increase its independence. A major psychiatric and psychological work must also be done. Solutions have been developed and tested for those patients.

A virtual reality system has been developed and tested with patients with schizophrenia. After interventions, they had significant higher cognitive function, better self-esteem, and better work performance compared with patients receiving conventional and traditional care (Tsang and Man 2013).

The same findings were found in an almost similar study on the use of cognitive rehabilitation techniques based on computational methods for improving cognitive functions and working capacity (Lee 2013b).

Interventions to promote and encourage social skills are beneficial for patient with psychotic disorders. However, in clinics it is difficult to perform this kind of intervention with patients. The virtual reality could be used to facilitate this kind of intervention. Current studies tend to show that virtual reality training could be effective to increase the social functions and interactions of these patients in activities of daily living (Rus-Calafell et al. 2014).

Finally, it has been demonstrated that the behavior of the patients during different tasks of virtual navigation was different compared to healthy individuals. The use of games might therefore be used in the future as a diagnostic tool to manage and select the best therapeutic interventions.

4.9.5   Down Syndrome

Down syndrome (trisomy 21) induces a significant cognitive delay and various mus-culoskeletal system disorders. After a 24 weeks rehabilitation program (2 sessions per week) using the video games, a significant increase in sensorimotor functions (motor control, visual skills, and sensory integration) was observed in the patients playing games compared to a group with conventional sessions of occupational therapy. (Wuang et al. 2011).

4.9.6   Mild Cognitive Impairment

Video games can also be used with patients with mild cognitive impairment to improve both cognitive and motor functions. One of the advantages highlighted by the authors is that training with video games at the home could solve some barriers to rehabilitation (access to care, cost) and allow the patient to perform moderate physical activities. Such solutions enable people to stay more active (Padala et al. 2011).

In another study, 40 children with developmental delays have benefited from intervention using video games. Significant improvements in balance and grip strength were observed compared to the control group (Salem et al. 2012). It has also been demonstrated that a 6 weeks training program (3 sessions per week) was effective to increase aerobic capacity (endurance) of patients with developmental disorders and coordination issues.

4.9.7   Alzheimer's Disease

Video games were also tested with patients with another important cognitive disor-ders: Alzheimer's disease. After a period of 12 weeks of training, the authors dem-onstrated that despite the cognitive and motor disorders associated with the disease Alzheimer's patients were still able to play (Padala et al. 2011).

Of course depending on the cognitive abilities and the severity of the disease, these patients were either able to play the games directly and train during the first session or some sessions were required before they can understand how to play.

In most cases, patients were satisfied with this activity and wished to continue with the game after the study (Boulay et al. 2011).

4.9.8   Pulmonary Diseases

In case of obstructive pulmonary diseases (asthma, chronic obstructive pulmonary disease [COPD]), management consists in bronchial decluttering, respiratory reha-bilitation as well as a progressive retraining. Active video games may play a positive role in this recovery.

The use of commercial video games in patients with cystic fibrosis showed that playing with these games provided a level of moderate intensity physical activity in children (O'Donovan et al. 2013) and high intensity in adults (Holmes et al. 2013).

A feasibility study was conducted with 32 patients admitted in pulmonary rehabilitation service. After 4 weeks of treatment with 3 sessions per week, the authors found that use of the games was safe for the patients and allows them to practice at a moderate physical activity level during the rehabilitation session (Wardini et al. 2013).

Using video games also seems to have a direct positive effect on lung function. After a 12 week program (5 sessions per week), it has been shown that the patient had a significant increase in expiratory strength and endurance as well as for some psychological parameters (quality of life and emotions) (Albores et al. 2013).

Finally, specific games were developed to train expiratory capacity with COPD patients. These games are controlled by a spirometer. After a training period of 2 weeks, the results of all pulmonary measurements were increased. However, it is not clear whether this increase is due to clinical improvement in lung function or a habituation of the spirometry (Bingham et al. 2012).

4.9.9 Diabetes

Diabetes is defined by excessive glucose concentration in the blood (blood sugar). There is a lack of insulin production in the pancreas in the case of type I diabetes; in the case of type II diabetes, insulin is produced normally but there is a resistance of muscle cells, fat tissues, and liver to this hormone. This resistance is in most cases due to modern lifestyle: bad eating habits (fast acting sugar) and not enough physical activity. We already discussed that the games could be used to educate patients about the problem of diabetes and glycemic control (Sect. 3.3.2). For patients with type II diabetes, it is important to promote regular physical activity and modify the alimentation. Serious games can help with this. An extensive study with 220 patients showed that after 12 weeks of daily training using the Nintendo Wii Fit there was a significant decrease of the blood parameters (glycated hemoglobin, fasting blood sugar level), weight, and BMI. The general level of physical activity was also significantly increased. Another interesting point to note is when patients are more physically active they also have a better quality of life and mental state (decrease depression and increase self-esteem) (Kempf and Martin 2013).

This study demonstrates, once again, the importance of promoting physical activity not only for the direct physical benefits it provides but also for the many related positive psychological aspects (Lee and Shin 2013).

4.9.10 Urinary Incontinence

Urinary incontinence is the uncontrollable and involuntary loss of urine. Because of the constitution of the pelvic floor and the constraints on it during pregnancy or childbirth, these disorders are much more common in women than in men. Coupled to preventive exercises (e.g., hypopressive abdominal exercises), the rehabilitation exercises (strengthening of the pelvic floor muscles and proprioception) are key pieces of the urinary incontinence management.

Dance video game was tested with patients presenting urinary incontinence. These games were used as functional rehabilitation tool (strength, proprioception, mobility) in combination with the conventional rehabilitation exercises for the pelvic floor muscles (contraction and proprioception). After a 12 week intervention (one session per week), the 24 patients included in the study showed a decrease in the amount of urine leakage, an increase in quality of life and increased adherence to treatment (Elliott et al. 2015).

Another study showed that training with video games is possible to increase the executive functions of these patients and the walking ability in dual-task situation. The authors have shown not only a decrease in urinary incontinence but also an improvement of walking in dual-task condition, these factors indicate a decreased risk of falling that, as we have seen, can be particularly dangerous and debilitating for older patients (Fraser et al. 2014).

4.9.11 Pain Management

Pain is the most common complaint in medical consultation.

Several approaches can be used to integrate the games in pain management program.

The first is that games can be used for educational purposes to explain the disease, the treatment, or adverse side effects inherent of it. We have already presented the case of the "Captain Novolin" game for diabetic patients (Brown et al. 1997) and the play "Re-Mission" for cancer patients (Beale et al. 2007). We also saw the importance of education and information on issues related to overweight and obesity.

Pain, especially chronic pain, remains a relatively poor and poorly understood process. Therefore, patients are asking many questions. Health professionals are not always present and available to respond. Thus, "virtual coaches" have been developed (explanatory videos, texts, videos) to answer the questions of the patients and help them.

These virtual systems have proven their efficacy in the treatment of chronic pain associated with osteoarthritis in the elderly. This tool appears to be a feasible solution to increase the dialogue on pain management between patient and therapist (McDonald et al. 2013).

Finally, the third approach is to create a distraction phenomenon in patients when performing painful procedures. The challenge for developers is to create games in which the patients won't move but will be immersed enough in order to not feel pain.

Such solutions have been developed for young children going to the dentist. There was a significant decrease in pain perception and anxiety with the use of virtual reality glasses and games during dental treatment (Asl Aminabadi et al. 2012). Another particularly painful condition is the treatment of severe burns. Virtual reality and serious games can be used to reduce pain during wound cleaning. The results seem to be maintained over time; in fact, after 3 or 4 days there is always a positive effect on pain during care (Faber et al. 2013).

References

Ackerman PL, Kanfer R, Calderwood C. Use it or lose it? Wii brain exercise practice and reading for domain knowledge. Psychol Aging. 2010;25(4):753–66.

Adamo KB, Rutherford JA, Goldfield GS. Effects of interactive video game cycling on overweight and obese adolescent health. Appl Physiol Nutr Metab. 2010;35(6):805–15.

Agmon M, Perry CK, Phelan E, Demiris G, Nguyen HQ. A pilot study of Wii fit exergames to improve balance in older adults. J Geriatr Phys Ther. 2011;34(4):161–7.

Akhutina T, Foreman N, Krichevets A, Matikka L, Narhi V, Pylaeva N, Vahakuopus J. Improving spatial functioning in children with cerebral palsy using computerized and traditional game tasks. Disabil Rehabil. 2003;25(24):1361–71.

Alahakone AU, Senanayake S, Arosha M. A real-time system with assistive feedback for postural control in rehabilitation. IEEE/ASME Trans Mechatron. 2010;15:226–33.

Albores J, Marolda C, Haggerty M, Gerstenhaber B, Zuwallack R. The use of a home exercise program based on a computer system in patients with chronic obstructive pulmonary disease. J Cardiopulm Rehabil Prev. 2013;33(1):47–52.

Al Saif AA, Alsenany S. Effects of interactive games on motor performance in children with spastic cerebral palsy. J Phys Ther Sci. 2015;27(6):2001–3.

Andrysek J, Klejman S, Steinnagel B, Torres-Moreno R, Zabjek KF, Salbach NM, Moody K. Preliminary evaluation of a commercially available videogame system as an adjunct therapeutic intervention for improving balance among children and adolescents with lower limb amputations. Arch Phys Med Rehabil. 2012;93(2):358–66.

Anguera JA, Baccanfuso J, Rintoul JL, Al-Hashimi O, Faraji F, Janowich J, Kong E, Larraburo Y, Rolle C, Johnston E, Gazzaley A. Video game training enhances cognitive control in older adults. Nature. 2013;501(7465):97–101.

Asl Aminabadi N, Erfanparast L, Sohrabi A, Ghertasi Oskouei S, Naghili A. The impact of virtual reality distraction on pain and anxiety during dental treatment in 4-6 year-old children: a randomized controlled clinical trial. J Dent Res Dent Clin Dent Prospects. 2012;6(4):117–24.

Baltaci G, Harput G, Haksever B, Ulusoy B, Ozer H. Comparison between Nintendo Wii fit and conventional rehabilitation on functional performance outcomes after hamstring anterior cruciate ligament reconstruction: prospective, randomized, controlled, double-blind clinical trial. Knee Surg Sports Traumatol Arthrosc. 2013;21(4):880–7.

Bamidis PD, Fissler P, Papageorgiou SG, Zilidou V, Konstantinidis EI, Billis AS, Romanopoulou E, Karagianni M, Beratis I, Tsapanou A, Tsilikopoulou G, Grigoriadou E, Ladas A, Kyrillidou A, Tsolaki A, Frantzidis C, Sidiropoulos E, Siountas A, Matsi S, Papatriantafyllou J, Margioti E, Nika A, Schlee W, Elbert T, Tsolaki M, Vivas AB, Kolassa IT. Gains in cognition through combined cognitive and physical training: the role of training dosage and severity of neurocognitive disorder. Front Aging Neurosci. 2015;7:152.

Bao X, Mao Y, Lin Q, Qiu Y, Chen S, Li L, Cates RS, Zhou S, Huang D. Mechanism of Kinect-based virtual reality training for motor functional recovery of upper limbs after subacute stroke. Neural Regen Res. 2013;8(31):2904–13.

Barcala L, Grecco LA, Colella F, Lucareli PR, Salgado AS, Oliveira CS. Visual biofeedback balance training using wii fit after stroke: a randomized controlled trial. J Phys Ther Sci. 2013;25(8):1027–32.

Bateni H. Changes in balance in older adults based on use of physical therapy vs the Wii fit gaming system: a preliminary study. Physiotherapy. 2012;98(3):211–6.

Beale IL, Kata PM, Marin-Bowling VM, Guthrie N, Cole SW. Improvement in cancer-related knowledge following use of a psychoeducational video game for adolescent and young adults with cancer. J Adolesc Health. 2007;41(3):263–70.

Bieryla KA, Dold NM. Feasibility of Wii fit training to improve clinical measures of balance in older adults. Clin Interv Aging. 2013;8:775–81.

Biffi A, Anderson CD, Battee TW, Ayres AM, Greenberg SM, Viswanathan A, Rosand J. Association between blood pressure control and risk of recurrent intracerebral haemorrhage. JAMA. 2015;314(9):904–12.

Bingham PM, Lahiri T, Ashikaga T. Pilot trial of spirometer games for airway clearance practice in cystic fibrosis. Respir Care. 2012;57(8):1278–84.

Bonnechère B, Jansen B, Omelina L, Van Sint Jan S. The use of commercial video games in rehabilitation: a systematic review. Int J Rehabil Res. 2016;39(4):277–90.

Bonnechère B, Omelina L, Jansen B, Van Sint Jan S. Balance improvement after physical therapy training using specially developed serious games for cerebral palsy children: preliminary results. Disabil Rehabil. 2015;18:1–4.

Botella C, Garcia-Palacios A, Vizcaíno Y, Herrero R, Baños RM, Belmonte MA. Virtual reality in the treatment of fibromyalgia: a pilot study. Cyberpsychol Behav Soc Netw. 2013;16(3):215–23.

Boulay M, Benveniste S, Boespflug S, Jouvelot P, Rigaud AS. A pilot usability study of MINWii, a music therapy game for demented patients. Technol Health Care. 2011;19(4):233–46.

Bower KJ, Clark RA, McGinley JL, Martin CL, Miller KJ. Clinical feasibility of the Nintendo Wii™ for balance training post-stroke: a phase II randomized controlled trial in an inpatient setting. Clin Rehabil. 2014;28(9):912–23.

Bower KJ, Louie J, Landesrocha Y, Seedy P, Gorelik A, Bernhardt J. Clinical feasibility of interactive motion-controlled games for stroke rehabilitation. J Neuroeng Rehabil. 2015;12:63.

Brichetto G, Spallarossa P, de Carvalho ML, Battaglia MA. The effect of Nintendo® Wii® on balance in people with multiple sclerosis: a pilot randomized control study. Mult Scler. 2013;19(9):1219–21.

Brown SJ, Lieberman DA, Germeny BA, Fan YC, Wilson DM, Pasta DJ. Educational video game for juvenile diabetes: results of a controlled trial. Med Inform (Lond). 1997;22(1):77–89.

Byl N, Zhang W, Coo S, Tomizuka M. Clinical impact of gait training enhanced with visual kinematic biofeedback: patients with parkinson's disease and patients stable post stroke. Neuropsychologia. 2015;79:332–43.

Caudron S, Guerraz M, Eusebio A, Gros J-P, Azulay J-P, Vaugoyeau M. Evaluation of a visual biofeedback on the postural control in parkinson's disease. Neurophys Clin Neurophysiol. 2014;44:77–86.

Celinder D, Peoples H. Stroke patients' experiences with Wii sports® during inpatient rehabilitation. Scand J Occup Ther. 2012;19(5):457–63.

Chan TC, Chan F, Shea YF, Lin OY, Luk JK, Chan FH. Interactive virtual reality Wii in geriatric day hospital: a study to assess its feasibility, acceptability and efficacy. Geriatr Gerontol Int. 2012;12(4):714–21.

Chao YY, Scherer YK, Montgomery CA, Wu YW, Lucke KT. Physical and psychosocial effects of Wii fit exergames use in assisted living residents: a pilot study. Clin Nurs Res. 2015;24(6):589–603.

Chao YY, Scherer YK, Wu YW, Lucke KT, Montgomery CA. The feasibility of an intervention combining self-efficacy theory and Wii fit exergames in assisted living residents: a pilot study. Geriatr Nurs. 2013;34(5):377–82.

Chen CL, Chen CY, Liaw MY, Chung CY, Wang CJ, Hong WH. Efficacy of home-based virtual cycling training on bone mineral density in ambulatory children with cerebral palsy. Osteoporos Int. 2013;24(4):1399–406.

Chen CL, Hong WH, Cheng HY, Liaw MY, Chung CY, Chen CY. Muscle strength enhancement following home-based virtual cycling training in ambulatory children with cerebral palsy. Res Dev Disabil. 2012a;33(4):1087–94.

Chen JL, Weiss S, Heyman MB, Cooper B, Lustig RH. The efficacy of the web-based childhood obesity prevention program in Chinese-American adolescents (qeb ABC study). J Adolesc Health. 2011;49(2):148–54.

Chen MH, Huang LL, Lee CF, Hsieh CL, Lin YC, Liu H, Chen MI, Lu WS. A controlled pilot trial of two commercial video games for rehabilitation of arm function after stroke. Clin Rehabil. 2015;29(7):674–82.

Chen PY, Wei SH, Hsieh WL, Cheen JR, Chen LK, Kao CL. Lower limb power rehabilitation (LLPR) using interactive video game for improvement of balance function in older people. Arch Gerontol Geriatr. 2012b;55(3):677–82.

Chen YP, Kang LJ, Chuang TY, Doong JL, Lee SJ, Tsai MW, Jeng SF, Sung WH. Use of virtual reality to improve upper-extremity control in children with cerebral palsy: a single-subject design. Phys Ther. 2007;87(11):1441–57.

Chiu HC, Ada L, Lee HM. Upper limb training using Wii sports resort for children with hemiplegic cerebral palsy: a randomized, single-blind trial. Clin Rehabil. 2014;28(10):1015–24.

Cho KH, Lee KJ, Song CH. Virtual-reality balance training with a video-game system improves dynamic balance in chronic stroke patients. Tohoku J Exp Med. 2012;228(1):69–74.

Cho GH, Hwangbo G, Shin HS. The effects of virtual reality-based balance training on balance of the elderly. J Phys Ther Sci. 2014;26(4):615–7.

Choi JH, Han EY, Kim BR, Kim SM, Im SH, Lee SY, Hyun CW. Effectiveness of commercial gaming-based virtual reality movement therapy on functional recovery of upper extremity in subacute stroke patients. Ann Rehabil Med. 2014;38(4):485–93.

Christison A, Khan HA. Exergaming for health: a community-based pediatric weight management program using active video gaming. Clin Pediatr (Phila). 2012;51(4):382–8.

Cone BL, Levy SS, Goble DJ. Wii fit exer-game training improves sensory weighting and dynamic balance in healthy young adults. Gait Posture. 2015;41(2):711–5.

Cuthbert JP, Staniszewski K, Hays K, Gerber D, Natale A, O'Dell D. Virtual reality-based therapy for the treatment of balance deficits in patients receiving inpatient rehabilitation for traumatic brain injury. Brain Inj. 2014;28(2):181–8.

da Silva Ribeiro NM, Ferraz DD, Pedreira É, Pinheiro Í, da Silva Pinto AC, Neto MG, Dos Santos LR, Pozzato MG, Pinho RS, Masruha MR. Virtual rehabilitation via Nintendo Wii® and conventional physical therapy effectively treat post-stroke hemiparetic patients. Top Stroke Rehabil. 2015;22(4):299–305.

Daniel K. Wii-hab for pre-frail older adults. Rehabil Nurs. 2012;37(4):195–201.

de Kloet AJ, Berger MA, Verhoeven IM, van Stein CK, Vlieland TP. Gaming supports youth with acquired brain injury? A pilot study. Brain Inj. 2012;26(7–8):1021–9.

de Mello Monteiro CB, Massetti T, da Silva TD, van der Kamp J, de Abreu LC, Leone C, Savelsbergh GJ. Transfer of motor learning from virtual to natural environments in individuals with cerebral palsy. Res Dev Disabil. 2014;35(10):2430–7.

dos Santos Mendes FA, Pompeu JE, Modenesi Lobo A, da Silva KG, Oliveira Tde P, Peterson Zomignani A, Pimentel Piemonte ME. Motor learning, retention and transfer after virtualrealitybased training in Parkinson's disease—effect of motor and cognitive demands of games: a longitudinal, controlled clinical study. Physiotherapy. 2012;98(3):217–23.

Dowling GA, Hone R, Brown C, Mastick J, Melnick M. Feasibility of adapting a classroom balance training program to a video game platform for people with Parkinson's disease. Telemed J E Health. 2013;19(4):298–304.

Doyle AC, Goldschmidt A, Huang C, Winzelberg AJ, Taylor CB, Wilfley DE. Reduction of overweight and eating disorder symptoms via the internet in adolescents: a randomized controlled trial. J Adolesc Health. 2008;43(2):172–9.

Duque G, Boersma D, Loza-Diaz G, Hassan S, Suarez H, Geisinger D, Suriyaarachchi P, Sharma A, Demontiero O. Effects of balance training using a virtual-reality system in older fallers. Clin Interv Aging. 2013;8:257–63.

Elliott V, de Bruin ED, Dumoulin C. Virtual reality rehabilitation as a treatment approach for older women with mixed urinary incontinence: a feasibility study. Neurourol Urodyn. 2015;34(3):236–43.

Esculier JF, Vaudrin J, Bériault P, Gagnon K, Tremblay LE. Home-based balance training programme using Wii fit with balance board for Parkinsons's disease: a pilot study. J Rehabil Med. 2012;44(2):144–50.

Esculier JF, Vaudrin J, Tremblay LE. Corticomotor excitability in Parkinson's disease during observation, imagery and imitation of action: effects of rehabilitation using Wii fit and comparison to healthy controls. J Parkinsons Dis. 2014;4(1):67–75.

Faber AW, Patterson DR, Bremer M. Repeated use of immersive virtual reality therapy to control pain during wound dressing changes in pediatric and adult burn patients. J Burn Care Res. 2013;34(5):563–8.

Feltz DL, Irwin B, Kerr N. Two-player partnered exergame for obesity prevention: using discrepancy in players' abilities as a strategy to motivate physical activity. J Diabetes Sci Technol. 2012;6(4):820–7.

Fernandes AB, Passos JO, Brito PD, Campos TF. Comparison of the immediate effects of the training with a virtual reality game in stroke patients according side brain injury. NeuroRehabilitation. 2014;35(1):39–45.

Franco C, Fleury A, Guméry P-Y, Diot B, Demongeot J, Vuillerme N. Ibalance-abf: a smartphone-based audio-biofeedback balance system. IEEE Trans Biomed Eng. 2013;60:211–5.

Franco JR, Jacobs K, Inzerillo C, Kluzik J. The effect of the Nintendo Wii fit and exercise in improving balance and quality of life in community dwelling elders. Technol Health Care. 2012;20(2):95–115.

Fraser SA, Elliott V, de Bruin ED, Bherer L, Dumoulin C. The effects of combining videogame dancing and pelvic floor training to improve dual-task gait and cognition in women with mixedurinary incontinence. Games Health J. 2014;3(3):172–8.

Fu AS, Gao KL, Tung AK, Tsang WW, Kwan MM. Effectiveness of Exergaming training in reducing risk and incidence of falls in frail older adults with a history of falls. Arch Phys Med Rehabil. 2015;96(12):2096–102.

Fung V, Ho A, Shaffer J, Chung E, Gomez M. Use of Nintendo Wii fit™ in the rehabilitation of outpatients following total knee replacement: a preliminary randomised controlled trial. Physiotherapy. 2012;98(3):183–8.

Galna B, Jackson D, Schofield G, McNaney R, Webster M, Barry G, Mhiripiri D, Balaam M, Olivier P, Rochester L. *Retraining function in people with Parkinson's disease using the Microsoft kinect: game design and pilot testing.* J Neuroeng Rehabil. 2014;11:60.

Garcia AP, Ganaça MM, Cusin FS, Tomaz A, Ganança FF, Caovilla HH. Vestibular rehabilitation with a virtual reality in Ménière's disease. Braz J Otorhinolaryngol. 2013;79(3):366–74.

Giansanti D, Dozza M, Chiari L, Maccioni G, Cappello A. Energetic assessment of trunk postural modifications induced by a wearable audio-biofeedback system. Med Eng Phys. 2009;31:48–54.

Gioftsidou A, Vernadakis N, Malliou P, Batzios S, Sofokleous P, Antoniou P, Kouli O, Tsapralis K, Godolias G. Typical balance exercises or exergames for balance improvement? J Back Musculoskelet Rehabil. 2013;26(3):299–305. doi:10.3233/BMR-130384.

Golomb MR, McDonald BC, Warden SJ, Yonkman J, Saykin AJ, Shirley B, Huber M, Rabin B, Abdelbaky M, Nwosu ME, Barkat-Masih M, Burdea GC. In-home virtual reality videogame telerehabilitation in adolescents with hemiplegic cerebral palsy. Arch Phys Med Rehabil. 2010;91(1):1–8.e1.

Gonçalves GB. Using the Nintendo® Wii fit™ plus platform in the sensorimotor training of freezing of gait in Parkinson's disease. Arq Neuropsiquiatr. 2013;71(10):828.

Gordon C, Roopchand-Martin S, Gregg A. Potential of the Nintendo Wii™ as a rehabilitation tool for children with cerebral palsy in a developing country: a pilot study. Physiotherapy. 2012;98(3):238–42.

Graves LE, Ridgers ND, Atkinson G, Stratton G. The effect of active video gaming on children's physical activity, behavior preferences and body composition. Pediatr Exerc Sci. 2010;22(4):535–46.

Green D, Wilson PH. Use of virtual reality in rehabilitation of movement in children with hemiplegia—a multiple case study evaluation. Disabil Rehabil. 2012;34(7):593–604.

Grewal GS, Sayeed R, Schwenk M, Bharara M, Menzies R, Talal TK, Armstrong DG, Najafi B. Balance rehabilitation: promoting the role of virtual reality in patients with diabetic peripheral neuropathy. J Am Podiatr Med Assoc. 2013;103(6):498–507.

Grewal GS, Schwenk M, Lee-Eng J, Parvaneh S, Bharara M, Menzies RA, Talal TK, Armstrong DG, Najafi B. Sensor-based interactive balance training with visual joint movement feedback for improving postural stability in diabetics with peripheral neuropathy: a randomized controlled trial. Gerontology. 2015;61(6):567–74.

Griffin M, McCormick D, Taylor MJ, Shawis T, Impson R. Using the Nintendo Wii as an intervention in a falls prevention group. J Am Geriatr Soc. 2012;60(2):385–7.

Gschwind YJ, Eichberg S, Marston HR, Ejupi A, Rosario H, Kroll M, Drobics M, Annegarn J, Wieching R, Lord SR, Aal K, Delbaere K. ICT-based system to predict and prevent falls (iStoppFalls): study protocol for an international multicenter randomized controlled trial. BMC Geriatr. 2014;14:91.

Gschwind YJ, Schoene D, Lord SR, Ejupi A, Valenzuela T, Aal K, Woodbury A, Delbaere K. The effect of sensor-based exercise at home on functional performance associated with fall risk in older people—a comparison of two exergame interventions. Eur Rev Aging Phys Act. 2015;12:11.

Guderian B, Borreson LA, Sletten LE, Cable K, Stecker TP, Probst MA, Dalleck LC. The cardiovascular and metabolic responses to Wii Fit video game playing in middle-aged and older adults. J Sports Med Phys Fitness. 2010;50:436–42.

Gutiérrez RO, Galán Del Río F, Cano de la Cuerda R, Alguacil Diego IM, González RA, Page JC. A telerehabilitation program by virtual reality-video games improves balance and postural control in multiple sclerosis patients. NeuroRehabilitation. 2013;33(4):545–54.

Halická Z, Lobotková J, Bučková K, Hlavačka F. Effectiveness of different visual biofeedback signals for human balance improvement. Gait Posture. 2014;39(1):410–4.

Harris K, Reid DM. The influence of virtual reality play on children's motivation. Can J Occup Ther. 2005;72(1):21–9.

Herrero R, García-Palacios A, Castilla D, Molinari G, Botella C. Virtual reality for the induction of positive emotions in the treatment of fibromyalgia: a pilot study over acceptability, satisfaction, and the effect of virtual reality on mood. Cyberpsychol Behav Soc Netw. 2014;17(6):379–84.

Herz NB, Mehta SH, Sethi KD, Jackson P, Hall P, Morgan JC. Nintendo Wii rehabilitation ("Wii-hab") provides benefits in Parkinson's disease. Parkinsonism Relat Disord. 2013;19(11):1039–42.

Heuschling A, Gazagnes MD, Hatem SM. Accident Vasculaire Cérébral: de la prise en charge précoce à la rééducation. Rev Med Brux. 2013;34(4):205–10.

Höchsmann C, Zürcher N, Stamm A, Schmidt-Trucksäss A. Cardiorespiratory exertion while playing video game exercises in elderly individuals with type 2 diabetes. Clin J Sport Med. 2016;26(4):326–31.

Holmes H, Wood J, Jenkins S, Winship P, Lunt D, Bostock S, Hill K. Xbox Kinect™ represents high intensity exercise for adults with cystic fibrosis. J Cyst Fibros. 2013;12(6):604–8.

Hsu JK, Thibodeau R, Wong SJ, Zukiwsky D, Cecile S, Walton DM. A "Wii" bit of fun: the effects of adding Nintendo Wii(®) bowling to a standard exercise regimen for residents of long-term care with upper extremity dysfunction. Physiother Theory Pract. 2011;27(3):185–93.

Hung JW, Chou CX, Hsieh YW, Wu WC, Yu MY, Chen PC, Chang HF, Ding SE. Randomized comparison trial of balance training by using exergaming and conventional weight-shift therapy in patients with chronic stroke. Arch Phys Med Rehabil. 2014;95(9):1629–37.

Hung SH, Hwang SL, Su MJ, et al. An evaluation of a weight-loss program incorporating E-learning for obese junior high school students. Telemed J E Health. 2008;14(8):783–92.

Hurkmans HL, Ribbers GM, Streur-Kranenburg MF, Stam HJ, van den Berg-Emons RJ. Energy expenditure in chronic stroke patients playing Wii sports: a pilot study. J Neuroeng Rehabil. 2011;8:38.

Hurkmans HL, van den Berg-Emons RJ, Stam HJ. Energy expenditure in adults with cerebral palsy playing Wii sports. Arch Phys Med Rehabil. 2010;91(10):1577–81.

Iosa M, Morone G, Fusco A, Castagnoli M, Fusco FR, Pratesi L, Paolucci S. Leap motion controlled videogame-based therapy for rehabilitation of elderly patients with subacutestroke: a feasibility pilot study. Top Stroke Rehabil. 2015;22(4):306–16.

Jago R, Baranowski T, Baranowski JC, et al. Fit for life boy scout badge: outcome evaluation of a troop and internet intervention. Prev Med. 2006;42(3):181–7.

Jannink MJ, van der Wilden GJ, Navis DW, Visser G, Gussinklo J, Ijzerman M. A low-cost video game applied for training of upper extremity function in children with cerebral palsy: a pilot study. Cyberpsychol Behav. 2008;11(1):27–32.

Janssen M, Stokroos R, Aarts J, van Lummel R, Kingma H. Salient and placebo vibrotactile feedback are equally effective in reducing sway in bilateral vestibular loss patients. Gait Posture. 2010;31:213–7.

Jaume-i-Capó A, Martínez-Bueso P, Moyà-Alcover B, Varona J. Interactive rehabilitation system for improvement of balance therapies in people with cerebral palsy. IEEE Trans Neural Syst Rehabil Eng. 2014;22(2):419–27.

Jelsma D, Geuze RH, Mombarg R, Smits-Engelsman BC. The impact of Wii fit intervention on dynamic balance control in children with probable developmental coordination disorder and balance problems. Hum Mov Sci. 2014;33:404–18.

Jelsma J, Pronk M, Ferguson G, Jelsma-Smit D. The effect of the Nintendo Wii fit on balance control and gross motor function of children with spastic hemiplegic cerebral palsy. Dev Neurorehabil. 2013;16(1):27–37.

Johnston JD, Massey AP, Marker-Hoffman RL. Using an alternate reality game to increase physical activity and decrease obesity risk of college students. J Diabetes Sci Technol. 2012;6(4):828–38.

Jones M, Luce KH, Osborne MI, et al. Randomized, controlled trial of an internetfacilitated intervention for reducing binge eating and overweight in adolescents. Pediatrics. 2008;121(3):453–62.

Joo S, Shin D, Song C. The effects of game-based breathing exercise on pulmonary function in stroke patients: a preliminary study. Med Sci Monit. 2015;21:1806–11.

Jorgensen MG, Laessoe U, Hendriksen C, Nielsen OB, Aagaard P. Efficacy of Nintendo Wii training on mechanical leg muscle function and postural balance in community-dwelling older adults: a randomized controlled trial. J Gerontol A Biol Sci Med Sci. 2013;68(7):845–52.

Jung DI, Ko DS, Jeong MA. Kinematic effect of Nintendo Wii(TM) sports program exercise on obstacle gait in elderly women with falling risk. J Phys Ther Sci. 2015;27(5):1397–400.

Kafri M, Myslinski MJ, Gade VK, Deutsch JE. Energy expenditure and exercise intensity of interactive video gaming in individuals Poststroke. Neurorehabil Neural Repair. 2013;28(1):56–65.

Karahan AY, Tok F, Taşkın H, Kuçuksaraç S, Başaran A, Yıldırım P. *Effects of Exergames on Balance, Functional Mobility, and Quality of Life of Geriatrics Versus Home Exercise Programme: Randomized Controlled Study*. Cent Eur J Public Health. 2015;23(Suppl):S14–8.

Kempf K, Martin S. *Autonomous exercise game use improves metabolic control and quality of life in type 2 diabetes patients—a randomized controlled trial*. BMC Endocr Disord. 2013;13(1):57.

Keogh JWL, Power N, Wooller L, Lucas P, Whatman C. Physical and psychosocial function in residential aged care elders: effect of Nintendo Wii SportsGames. J Aging Phys Act. 2013;22(2):235–44.

Kim J, Son J, Ko N, Yoon B. Unsupervised virtual reality-based exercise program improves hip muscle strength and balance control in older adults: a pilot study. Arch Phys Med Rehabil. 2013;94(5):937–43.

Kim KJ, Heo M. Effects of virtual reality programs on balance in functional ankle instability. J Phys Ther Sci. 2015;27(10):3097–101.

Kim SS, Min WK, Kim JH, Lee BH. The effects of VR-based Wii fit yoga on physical function in middle-aged female LBP patients. J Phys Ther Sci. 2014;26(4):549–52.

Kiper P, Agostini M, Luque-Moreno C, Tonin P, Turolla A. Reinforced feedback in virtual environment for rehabilitation of upper extremity dysfunction after stroke: preliminary data from a randomized controlled trial. Biomed Res Int. 2014;2014:752128.

Kirshner S, Weiss PL, Tirosh E. Meal-maker: a virtual meal preparation environment for children with cerebral palsy. European Journal of Special Needs Education. 2011;26(3):323–36.

Lai CH, Peng CW, Chen YL, Huang CP, Hsiao YL, Chen SC. Effects of interactive video-game based system exercise on the balance of the elderly. Gait Posture. 2013;37(4):511–5.

Lamoth CJ, Caljouw SR, Postema K. Active video gaming to improve balance in the elderly. Stud Health Technol Inform. 2011;167:159–64.

Langhorne P, Bernhardt J, Kwakkel G. Stroke rehabilitation. Lancet. 2011;377:1693–702.

Lau PW, Liang Y, Lau EY, Choi CR, Kim CG, Shin MS. Evaluating physical and perceptual responses to exergames in Chinese children. Int J Environ Res Public Health. 2015;12(4):4018–30.

LeBlanc AG, Chaput JP, McFarlane A, Colley RC, Thivel D, Biddle SJ, Maddison R, Leatherdale ST, Tremblay MS. Active video games and health indicators in children and youth: a systematic review. PLoS One. 2013;8(6):e65351.

Lee G. Effects of training using video games on the muscle strength, muscle tone, and activities of daily living of chronic stroke patients. J Phys Ther Sci. 2013a;25(5):595–7.

Lee HY, Kim YL, Lee SM. Effects of virtual reality-based training and task-oriented training on balance performance in stroke patients. J Phys Ther Sci. 2015;27(6):1883–8.

Lee S, Shin S. Effectiveness of virtual reality using video gaming technology in elderly adults with diabetes mellitus. Diabetes Technol Ther. 2013;15(6):489–96.

Lee SJ, Chun MH. Combination transcranial direct current stimulation and virtual reality therapy for upper extremity training in patients with subacute stroke. Arch Phys Med Rehabil. 2014;95(3):431–8.

Lee WK. Effectiveness of computerized cognitive rehabilitation training on symptomatological, neuropsychological and work function in patients with schizophrenia. Asia Pac Psychiatry. 2013b;5(2):90–100.

Lehrl S, Gusinde J, Schulz-Drost S, Rein A, Schlechtweg PM, Jacob H, Krinner S, Gelse K, Pauser J, Brem MH. Advancement of physical process by mental activation: a prospective controlled study. J Rehabil Res Dev. 2012;49(8):1221–8.

Liao YY, Yang YR, Cheng SJ, Wu YR, Fuh JL, Wang RY. Virtual reality-based training to improve obstacle-crossing performance and dynamic balance in patients with Parkinson's disease. Neurorehabil Neural Repair. 2015;29(7):658–67.

Luna-Oliva L, Ortiz-Gutiérrez RM, Cano-de la Cuerda R, Piédrola RM, Alguacil-Diego IM, Sánchez-Camarero C, Martínez Culebras MD. Kinect Xbox 360 as a therapeutic modality for children with cerebral palsy in a school environment: a preliminary study. NeuroRehabilitation. 2013;33(4):513–21.

Lyons EJ, Tate DF, Komoski SE, Carr PM, Ward DS. Novel approaches to obesity prevention: effects of game enjoyment and game type on energy expenditure in active video games. J Diabetes Sci Technol. 2012;6(4):839–48.

Ma CZ-H, Wan AH-P, Wong DW-C, Zheng Y-P, Lee WC-C. A vibrotactile and plantar force measurement-based biofeedback system: paving the way towards wearable balance-improving devices. Sensors. 2015;15:31709–22.

Maddison R, Foley L, Ni Mhurchu C, Jiang Y, Jull A, Prapavessis H, Hohepa M, Rodgers A. Effects of active video games on body composition: a randomized controlled trial. Am J Clin Nutr. 2011;94(1):156–63.

Maillot P, Perrot A, Hartley A, Do MC. The braking force in walking: age-related differences and improvement in older adults with exergame training. J Aging Phys Act. 2014;22(4):518–26.

McDonald DD, Walsh S, Vergara C, Gifford T. Effect of a virtual pain coach on pain management discussions: a pilot study. Pain Manag Nurs. 2013;14(4):200–9.

McEwen D, Taillon-Hobson A, Bilodeau M, Sveistrup H, Finestone H. Virtual reality exercise improves mobility after stroke: an inpatient randomized controlled trial. Stroke. 2014;45(6):1853–5.

Meessen JM, Pisani S, Gambino ML, Bonarrigo D, van Schoor NM, Fozzato S, Cherubino P, Surace MF. Assessment of mortality risk in elderly patients after proximal femoral fracture. Orthopedics. 2014;37(2):e194–200.

Meldrum D, Herdman S, Moloney R, Murray D, Duffy D, Malone K, French H, Hone S, Conroy R, McConn-Walsh R. Effectiveness of conventional versus virtual reality based vestibular rehabilitation in the treatment of dizziness, gait and balance impairment in adults with unilateral peripheral vestibular loss: a randomised controlled trial. BMC Ear Nose Throat Disord. 2012;12:3.

Mhatre PV, Vilares I, Stibb SM, Albert MV, Pickering L, Marciniak CM, Kording K, Toledo S. Wii fit balance board playing improves balance and gait in Parkinson disease. PM R. 2013;5(9):769–77.

Mirelman A, Patritti BL, Bonato P, Deutsch JE. Effects of virtual reality training on gait biomechanics of individuals post-stroke. Gait Posture. 2010;31(4):433–7.

Mombarg R, Jelsma D, Hartman E. Effect of Wii-intervention on balance of children with poor motor performance. Res Dev Disabil. 2013;34(9):2996–3003.

Monteiro-Junior RS, de Souza CP, Lattari E, Rocha NB, Mura G, Machado S, da Silva EB. Wiiworkouts on chronic pain, physical capabilities and mood of older women: a randomized controlled double blind trial. CNS Neurol Disord Drug Targets. 2015;14(9):1157–64.

Morone G, Tramontano M, Iosa M, Shofany J, Iemma A, Musicco M, Paolucci S, Caltagirone C. The efficacy of balance training with video game-based therapy in subacute stroke patients: a randomized controlled trial. Biomed Res Int. 2014;2014:580861.

Mortensen J, Kristensen LQ, Brooks EP, Brooks AL. Women with fibromyalgia's experience with three motion-controlled video game consoles and indicators of symptom severity and performance of activities of daily living. Disabil Rehabil Assist Technol. 2015;10(1):61–6.

Mouawad MR, Doust CG, Max MD, McNulty PA. Wii-based movement therapy to promote improved upper extremity function post-stroke: a pilot study. J Rehabil Med. 2011;43(6):527–33.

Nacke LE, Nacke A, Lindley CA. Brain training for silver gamers: effects of age and game form on effectiveness, efficiency, self-assessment, and gameplay experience. Cyberpsychol Behav. 2009;12(5):493–9.

Nanhoe-Mahabier W, Allum J, Pasman E, Overeem S, Bloem B. The effects of vibrotactile biofeedback training on trunk sway in parkinson's disease patients. Parkinsonism Relat Disord. 2012;18:1017–21.

Naumann T, Kindermann S, Joch M, Munzert J, Reiser M. No transfer between conditions in balance training regimes relying on tasks with different postural demands: specificity effects of two different serious games. Gait Posture. 2015;41(3):774–9.

Neil A, Ens S, Pelletier R, Jarus T, Rand D. Sony PlayStation EyeToy elicits higher levels of movement than the Nintendo Wii: implications for stroke rehabilitation. Eur J Phys Rehabil Med. 2013;49(1):13–21.

Nicholson VP, McKean M, Lowe J, Fawcett C, Burkett B. Six weeks of unsupervised Nintendo Wii fit gaming is effective at improving balance in independent older adults. J Aging Phys Act. 2015;23(1):153–8.

Nilsagård YE, Forsberg AS, von Koch L. *Balance exercise for persons with multiple sclerosis using Wii games: a randomised, controlled multi-centre study.* Mult Scler. 2013;19(2):209–16.

Nitz JC, Kuys S, Isles R, Fu S. *Is the Wii Fit a new-generation tool for improving balance, health and well-being?* A pilot study. Climacteric. 2010;13(5):487–91.

O'Donovan C, Greally P, Canny G, McNally P, Hussey J. Active video games as an exercise tool for children with cystic fibrosis. J Cyst Fibros. 2013;13(3):341–6.

O'Donovan C, Roche EF, Hussey J. The energy cost of playing active video games in children with obesity and children of a healthy weight. Pediatr Obes. 2014;9(4):310–7.

Omiyale O, Crowell CR, Madhavan S. Effect of Wii-based balance training on corticomotor excitability post stroke. J Mot Behav. 2015;47(3):190–200.

Orihuela-Espina F, Fernández del Castillo I, Palafox L, Pasaye E, Sánchez-Villavicencio I, Leder R, Franco JH, Sucar LE. Neural reorganization accompanying upper limb motor rehabilitation from stroke with virtual reality-based gesture therapy. Top Stroke Rehabil. 2013;20(3):197–209.

Orsega-Smith E, Davis J, Slavish K, Gimbutas L. Wii fit balance intervention in communitydwelling older adults. Games Health J. 2012;1(6):431–5.

Ortiz-Gutiérrez R, Cano-de-la-Cuerda R, Galán-Del-Río F, Alguacil-Diego IM, PalaciosCeña D, Miangolarra-Page JC. A telerehabilitation program improves postural control in multiple sclerosis patients: a spanish preliminary study. Int J Environ Res Public Health. 2013;10(11):5697–710.

Padala KP, Padala PR, Burke WJ. Wii-fit as an adjunct for mild cognitive impairment: clinical perspectives. J Am Geriatr Soc. 2011;59(5):932–3.

Padala KP, Padala PR, Malloy TR, Geske JA, Dubbert PM, Dennis RA, Garner KK, Bopp MM, Burke WJ, Sullivan DH. Wii-fit for improving gait and balance in an assisted living facility: a pilot study. J Aging Res. 2012;2012:597573.

Palacios-Navarro G, García-Magariño I, Ramos-Lorente P. A Kinect-based system for lower limb rehabilitation in Parkinson's disease patients: a pilot study. J Med Syst. 2015;39(9):103.

Paquin K, Ali S, Carr K, Crawley J, McGowan C, Horton S. Effectiveness of commercial video gaming on fine motor control in chronic stroke within community-level rehabilitation. Disabil Rehabil. 2015;37(23):2184–91.

Park JH, Lee SH, Ko DS. *The Effects of the Nintendo Wii Exercise Program on Chronic Workrelated Low Back Pain in Industrial Workers.* J Phys Ther Sci. 2013;25(8):985–8.

Pau M, Coghe G, Corona F, Leban B, Marrosu MG, Cocco E. *Effectiveness and Limitations of Unsupervised Home-Based Balance Rehabilitation with NintendoWii in People with Multiple Sclerosis.* Biomed Res Int. 2015;2015:916478.

Peters DM, McPherson AK, Fletcher B, McClenaghan BA, Fritz SL. Counting repetitions: an observational study of video game play in people with chronic poststroke hemiparesis. J Neurol Phys Ther. 2013;37(3):105–11.

Pluchino A, Lee SY, Asfour S, Roos BA, Signorile JF. Pilot study comparing changes in postural control after training using a video game balance board program and 2 standard activity-based balance intervention programs. Arch Phys Med Rehabil. 2012;93(7):1138–46.

Pompeu JE, Arduini LA, Botelho AR, Fonseca MB, Pompeu SM, Torriani-Pasin C, Deutsch JE. Feasibility, safety and outcomes of playing Kinect adventures!™ for people with Parkinson's disease: a pilot study. Physiotherapy. 2014;100(2):162–8.

Pompeu JE, Mendes FA, Silva KG, Lobo AM, Oliveira Tde P, Zomignani AP, Piemonte ME. Effect of Nintendo Wii™-based motor and cognitive training on activities of daily living in patients with Parkinson's disease: a randomised clinical trial. Physiotherapy. 2012;98(3):196–204.

Prosperini L, Fortuna D, Giannì C, Leonardi L, Marchetti MR, Pozzilli C. Home-based balance training using the Wii balance board: a randomized, crossover pilot study in multiple sclerosis. Neurorehabil Neural Repair. 2013;27(6):516–25.

Quinn M. Introduction of active video gaming into the middle school curriculum as a school-based childhood obesity intervention. J Pediatr Health Care. 2013;27(1):3–12.

Rabin BA, Burdea GC, Roll DT, Hundal JS, Damiani F, Pollack S. Integrative rehabilitation of elderly stroke survivors: the design and evaluation of the BrightArm™. Disabil Rehabil Assist Technol. 2012 Jul;7(4):323–35.

Rajaratnam BS, Gui Kaien J, Lee Jialin K, Sweesin K, Sim Fenru S, Enting L, Ang Yihsia E, Keathwee N, Yunfeng S, Woo Yinghowe W, Teo SS. Does the inclusion of virtual reality games within conventional rehabilitation enhance balance retraining after a recent episode of stroke? Rehabil Res Pract. 2013;2013:649561.

Ramstrand N, Lygnegård F. Can balance in children with cerebral palsy improve through use of an activity promoting computer game? TechnolHealth Care. 2012;20:501–10.

Rand D, Givon N, Weingarden H, Nota A, Zeilig G. Eliciting upper extremity purposeful movements using video games: a comparison with traditional therapy for stroke rehabilitation. Neurorehabil Neural Repair. 2014;28(8):733–9.

Rendon AA, Lohman EB, Thorpe D, Johnson EG, Medina E, Bradley B. The effect of virtual reality gaming on dynamic balance in older adults. Age Ageing. 2012;41(4):549–52.

Reid DT, Campbell K. The use of virtual reality with children with cerebral palsy: a pilot randomized trial. Ther Recreat J. 2006;40(4):255–68.

Reid DT. Correlation of the pediatric volitional questionnaire with the test of playfulness In a virtual environment: the power of engagement. Early Child Dev Care. 2005;175(2):153–64.

Ritterband-Rosenbaum A, Christensen MS, Nielsen JB. Twenty weeks of computertraining improves sense of agency in children with spastic cerebral palsy. Res Dev Disabil. 2012;33(4):1227–34.

Robert M, Ballaz L, Hart R, Lemay M. Exercise intensity levels in children with cerebral palsy while playing with an active video game console. Phys Ther. 2013;93(8):1084–91.

Robinson J, Dixon J, Macsween A, van Schaik P, Martin D. The effects of exergaming on balance, gait, technology acceptance and flow experience in people with multiple sclerosis: a randomized controlled trial. BMC Sports Sci Med Rehabil. 2015;7:8.

Robles-Garcia V, Arias P, Sanmartin G, Espinosa N, Flores J, Grieve KL, Cudeiro J. Motor facilitation during realtime movement imitation in Parkinson's disease: a virtual reality study. Parkinsonism Relat Disrod. 2013;19(12):1123–9.

Roopchand-Martin S, McLean R, Gordon C, Nelson G. Balance training with Wii fit plus for community-dwelling persons 60 years and older. Games Health J. 2015;4(3):247–52.

Rosenberg D, Depp CA, Vahia IV, Reichstadt J, Palmer BW, Kerr J, Norman G, Jeste DV. Exergames for subsyndromal depression in older adults: a pilot study of a novel intervention. Am J Geriatr Psychiatry. 2010;18(3):221–6.

Rus-Calafell M, Gutiérrez-Maldonado J, Ribas-Sabaté J. A virtual reality-integrated program for improving social skills in patients with schizophrenia: a pilot study. J Behav Ther Exp Psychiatry. 2014;45(1):81–9.

Salem Y, Gropack SJ, Coffin D, Godwin EM. Effectiveness of a low-cost virtual reality system for children with developmental delay: a preliminary randomised single-blind controlled trial. Physiotherapy. 2012;98(3):189–95.

Samai AA, Martin-Schild S. Sex differences in predictors of ischemic stroke: current perspective. Vasc Health Risk Manag. 2015;11:427–36.

Sandlund M, Dock K, Häger CK, Waterworth EL. Motion interactive video games in home training for children with cerebral palsy: parents' perceptions. Disabil Rehabil. 2012;34(11):925–33.

Sandlund M, Domellöf E, Grip H, Rönnqvist L, Häger CK. Training of goal directed arm movements with motion interactive video games in children with cerebral palsy—a kinematic evaluation. Dev Neurorehabil. 2014;17(5):318–26.

Sandlund M, Waterworth EL, Häger C. Using motion interactive games to promote physical activity and enhance motor performance in children with cerebral palsy. Dev Neurorehabil. 2011;14(1):15–21.

Saposnik G, Teasell R, Mamdani M, Hall J, McIlroy W, Cheung D, Thorpe KE, Cohen LG, Bayley M, Stroke Outcome Research Canada (SORCan) Working Group. Effectiveness of virtual reality using Wii gaming technology in stroke rehabilitation: a pilot randomized clinical trial and proof of principle. Stroke. 2010;41(7):1477–84.

Schoene D, Lord SR, Delbaere K, Severino C, Davies TA, Smith ST. A randomized controlled pilot study of home-based step training in older people using videogame technology. PLoS One. 2013;8(3):e57734.

Schwenk M, Grewal GS, Honarvar B, Schwenk S, Mohler J, Khalsa DS, Najafi B. Interactive balance training integrating sensor-based visual feedback of movement performance: a pilot study in older adults. J Neuroeng Rehabil. 2014;11(1):164.

Sharan D, Ajeesh PS, Rameshkumar R, Mathankumar M, Paulina RJ, Manjula M. Virtual reality based therapy for post operative rehabilitation of children with cerebral palsy. Work. 2012;41(S1):3612–5.

Shin JH, Bog Park S, Ho JS. Effects of game-based virtual reality on health-related quality of life in chronic stroke patients: a randomized, controlled study. Comput Biol Med. 2015;63:92–8.

Shin JH, Ryu H, Jang SH. A task-specific interactive game-based virtual reality rehabilitation system for patients with stroke: a usability test and two clinical experiments. J Neuroeng Rehabil. 2014;11:32.

Shiner CT, Byblow WD, McNulty PA. Bilateral priming before wii-based movement therapy enhances upper limb rehabilitation and its retention after stroke: a case-controlled study. Neurorehabil Neural Repair. 2014;28(9):828–38.

Shiri S, Feintuch U, Lorber-Haddad A, Moreh E, Twito D, Tuchner-Arieli M, Meiner Z. Novel virtual reality system integrating online self-face viewing and mirror visual feedback for stroke rehabilitation: rationale and feasibility. Top Stroke Rehabil. 2012;19(4):277–86.

Sims J, Cosby N, Saliba EN, Hertel J, Saliba SA. Exergaming and static postural control in individuals with a history of lower limb injury. J Athl Train. 2013;48(3):314–25. doi:10.4085/1062-6050-48.2.04. Epub 2013 Feb 20

Şimşek TT, Çekok K. The effects of Nintendo Wii™-based balance and upper extremity training on activities of daily living and quality of life in patients with sub-acute stroke: a randomized controlled study. Int J Neurosci. 2016;126(12):1061–70.

Sin H, Lee G. Additional virtual reality training using Xbox Kinect in stroke survivors with hemiplegia. Am J Phys Med Rehabil. 2013;92(10):871–80.

Singh DK, Rajaratnam BS, Palaniswamy V, Pearson H, Raman VP, Bong PS. Participating in a virtual reality balance exercise program can reduce risk and fear of falls. Maturitas. 2012;73(3):239–43.

Singh DK, Rajaratnam BS, Palaniswamy V, Raman VP, Bong PS, Pearson H. Effects of balancefocused interactive games compared to therapeutic balance classes for older women. Climacteric. 2013;16(1):141–6.

Siriphorn A, Chamonchant D. Wii balance board exercise improves balance and lower limb muscle strength of overweight young adults. J Phys Ther Sci. 2015;27(1):41–6.

Song GB, Park EC. Effect of virtual reality games on stroke patients' balance, gait, depression, and interpersonal relationships. J Phys Ther Sci. 2015;27(7):2057–60.

Sparrer I, Duong Dinh TA, Ilgner J, Westhofen M. Vestibular rehabilitation using the Nintendo® Wii balance board—a user-friendly alternative for central nervous compensation. Acta Otolaryngol. 2013;133(3):239–45.

Staiano AE, Abraham AA, Calvert SL. Adolescent exergame play for weight loss and psychosocial improvement: a controlled physical activity intervention. Obesity (Silver Spring). 2013;21(3):598–601.

Staiano AE, Abraham AA, Calvert SL. Motivating effects of cooperative exergame play for overweight and obese adolescents. J Diabetes Sci Technol. 2012a;6(4):812–9.

Staiano AE, Abraham AA, Calvert SL. The Wii Club: gaming for weight loss in overweight and obese youth. Games Health J. 2012b;1(5):377–80.

Standen PJ, Threapleton K, Connell L, Richardson A, Brown DJ, Battersby S, Sutton CJ, Platts F. *Patients' use of a home-based virtual reality system to provide rehabilitation of the upper limb following stroke*. Phys Ther. 2015;95(3):350–9.

Stewart JC, Yeh SC, Jung Y, Yoon H, Whitford M, Chen SY, Li L, McLaughlin M, Rizzo A, Winstein CJ. Intervention to enhance skilled arm and hand movements after stroke: a feasibility study using a new virtual reality system. J Neuroeng Rehabil. 2007;4:21.

Stroebele N, Müller-Riemenschneider F, Nolte CH, Müller-Nordhorn J, Bockelbrink A, Willich SN. Knowledge of risk factors, and warning signs of stroke: a systematic review from gender perspective. Int J Strike. 2011;6(1):60–6.

Su H, Chang YK, Lin YJ, Chu IH. Effects of training using an active video game on agility and balance. J Sports Med Phys Fitness. 2015;55(9):914–21.

Subramaniam S, Wan-Ying Hui-Chan C, Bhatt T. A cognitive-balance control training paradigm using wii fit to reduce fall risk in chronic stroke survivors. J Neurol Phys Ther. 2014;38(4):216–25.

Sun TL, Lee CH. An impact study of the design of exergaming parameters on body intensity from objective and gameplay-based player experience perspectives, based on balance training exergame. PLoS One. 2013;8(7):e69471.

Sztum T, Betker AL, Moussavi Z, Desai A, Goodman V. Effects of an interactive computer game exercise regimen on balance impairment in frail community-dwelling older adults: a randomized controlled trial. Phys Ther. 2011 Oct;91(10):1449–62.

Szturm T, Polyzoi E, Marotta J, Srikesavan CS. An In-School-Based Program of combined fine motor exercise and educational activities for children with neurodevelopmental disorders. Games Health J. 2014;3(6):326–32.

Tarakci D, Ozdincler AR, Tarakci E, Tutuncuoglu F, Ozmen M. Wii-based balance therapy to improve balance function of children with cerebral palsy: a pilot study. J Phys Ther Sci. 2013;25(9):1123–7.

Taylor LM, Maddison R, Pfaeffli LA, Rawstorn JC, Gant N, Kerse NM. Activity and energy expenditure in older people playing active video games. Arch Phys Med Rehabil. 2012;93(12):2281–6.

Toril P, Reales JM, Ballesteros S. Video game training enhances cognition of older adults: a meta-analytic study. Psychol Aging. 2014;29(3):706–16.

Toulotte C, Toursel C, Olivier N. *Wii Fit® training vs. Adapted Physical Activities: which one is the most appropriate to improve the balance of independent senior subjects?* A randomized controlled study. Clin Rehabil. 2012;26(9):827–35.

Tripette J, Murakami H, Gando Y, Kawakami R, Sasaki A, Hanawa S, Hirosako A, Miyachi M. Home-based active video games to promote weight loss during the postpartum period. Med Sci Sports Exerc. 2014;46(3):472–8.

Trost SG, Sundal D, Foster GD, Lent MR, Vojta D. Effects of a pediatric weight management program with and without active video games a randomized trial. JAMA Pediatr. 2014;168(5):407–13.

Tsang MM, Man DW. A virtual reality-based vocational training system (VRVTS) for people with schizophrenia in vocational rehabilitation. Schizophr Res. 2013;144(1–3):51–62.

Tsekleves E, Paraskevopoulos IT, Warland A, Kilbride C. Development and preliminary evaluation of a novel low cost VR-based upper limb strokerehabilitation platform using Wii technology. Disabil Rehabil Assist Technol. 2014;13:1–10.

Turolla A, Dam M, Ventura L, Tonin P, Agostini M, Zucconi C, Kiper P, Cagnin A, Piron L. Virtual reality for the rehabilitation of the upper limb motor function after stroke: a prospective controlled trial. J Neuroeng Rehabil. 2013;10:85.

Ustinova KI, Leonard WA, Cassavaugh ND, Ingersoll CD. Development of a 3D immersive videogame to improve arm-postural coordination in patients with TBI. J Neuroeng Rehabil. 2011;8:61.

Uzor S, Baillie L, Skelton DA, Rowe PJ. Falls prevention advice and visual feedback to those at risk of falling: study protocol for a pilot randomized controlled trial. Trials. 2013;14:79.

van den Heuvel MR, Kwakkel G, Beek PJ, Berendse HW, Daffertshofer A, van Wegen EE. Effects of augmented visual feedback during balance training in Parkinson's disease: a pilot randomized clinical trial. Parkinsonism Relat Disord. 2014;20(12):1352–8.

van Gool CH, Penninx BW, Kempen GI, Rejeski WJ, Miller GD, van Eijk JT, Pahor M, Messier SP. Effects of exercise adherence on physical function among overweight older adults with knee osteoarthritis. Arthritis Rheum. 2005;53(1):24–32.

Vernadakis N, Derri V, Tsitskari E, Antoniou P. The effect of Xbox Kinect intervention on balance ability for previously injured young competitive male athletes: a preliminary study. Phys Ther Sport. 2014;15(3):148–55.

Viana RT, Laurentino GE, Souza RJ, Fonseca JB, Silva Filho EM, Dias SN, Teixeira-Salmela LF, Monte-Silva KK. Effects of the addition of transcranial direct current stimulation to virtual reality therapy after stroke: a pilot randomized controlled trial. NeuroRehabilitation. 2014;34(3):437–46.

Wagener TL, Fedele DA, Mignogna MR, Hester CN, Gillaspy SR. Psychological effects of dance-based group exergaming in obese adolescents. Pediatr Obes. 2012;7(5):e68–74.

Wall T, Feinn R, Chui K, Cheng MS. The effects of the Nintendo™ Wii fit on gait, balance, and quality of life in individuals with incomplete spinal cord injury. J Spinal Cord Med. 2015;38(6):777–83.

Wardini R, Dajczman E, Yang N, Baltzan M, Préfontaine D, Stathatos M, Marciano H, Watson S, Wolkove N. Using a virtual game system to innovate pulmonary rehabilitation: safety, adherence and enjoyment in severe chronic obstructive pulmonary disease. Can Respir J. 2013;20(5):357–61.

Williams B, Doherty NL, Bender A, Mattox H, Tibbs JR. The effect of nintendo wii on balance: a pilot study supporting the use of the wii in occupational therapy for the well elderly. Occup Ther Health Care. 2011;25(2–3):131–9.

Williams MA, Soiza RL, Jenkinson AM, Stewart A. Exercising with computers in later life (EXCELL) - pilot and feasibility study of the acceptability of the Nintendo® WiiFit in communitydwelling fallers. BMC Res Notes. 2010;3:238.

Winkels DG, Kotting AI, Temmink RA, Nijlant JM, Buurke JH. Wii™ habilitation of upper extremity function in children with cerebral palsy. An explorative study. Dev Neurorehabil. 2013;16(1):44–51.

Winter S, Autry A, Boyle C, Yeargin-Allsopp M. Trends in the prevalence of cerebral palsy in a population-based study. Pediatrics. 2002;110(6):1220–5.

White K, Schofield G, Kilding AE. Energy expended by boys playing active video games. J Sci Med Sports. 2011;14(2):130–4.

Wu YN, Hwang M, Ren Y, Gaebler-Spira D, Zhang LQ. Combined passive stretching and active movement rehabilitation of lower-limb impairments in children with cerebral palsy using a portable robot. Neurorehabil Neural Repair. 2011;25(4):378–85.

Wuang YP, Chiang CS, Su CY, Wang CC. Effectiveness of virtual reality using Wii gaming technology in children with down syndrome. Res Dev Disabil. 2011;32(1):312–21.

Wüest S, Borghese NA, Pirovano M, Mainetti R, van de Langenberg R, de Bruin ED. Usability and effects of an Exergame-based balance training program. Games Health J. 2014;3(2):106–14.

Yatar GI, Yildirim SA. Wii fit balance training or progressive balance training in patients with chronic stroke: a randomised controlled trial. J Phys Ther Sci. 2015;27(4):1145–51.

Yavuzer G, Senel A, Atay MB, Stam HJ. "Playstation eyetoy games" improve upper extremity-related motor functioning in subacute stroke: a randomized controlled clinical trial. Eur J Phys Rehabil Med. 2008;44(3):237–44.

Yong Joo L, Soon Yin T, Xu D, Thia E, Pei Fen C, Kuah CW, Kong KH. A feasibility study using interactive commercial off-the-shelf computer gaming in upper limb rehabilitation in patients after stroke. J Rehabil Med. 2010;42(5):437–41.

Yuen HK, Breland HL, Vogtle LK, Holthaus K, Kamen DL, Sword D. The process associated with motivation of a home-based Wii fit exercise program among sedentary African American women with systemic lupus erythematosus. Disabil Health J. 2013;6(1):63–8.

Yuen HK, Holthaus K, Kamen DL, Sword DO, Breland HL. Using Wii fit to reduce fatigue among African American women with systemic lupus erythematosus: a pilot study. Lupus. 2011;20(12):1293–9.

Zalecki T, Gorecka-Mazur A, Pietraszko W, Surowka AD, Novak P, Moskala M, Krygowska-Wajs A. Visual feedback training using WII fit improves balance in Parkinson's disease. Folia Med Cracov. 2013;53(1):65–78.

Zoccolillo L, Morelli D, Cincotti F, Muzzioli L, Gobbetti T, Paolucci S, Iosa M. Video-game based therapy performed by children with cerebral palsy: a cross-over randomized controlled trial and a cross-sectional quantitative measure of physical activity. Eur J Phys Rehabil Med. 2015;51(6):669–76.

Clinical and Practical Applications

5

Sometimes, you have to get to a point of total frustration before you'll be ready to make a big change. Don't wait for what anyone else should do but hasn't yet and likely won't. Instead, look for what is up to you and what you can do to change the situation for the better...even if i t means walking away entirely.

– Doe Zantamata

5.1 Body and Brain

The relation between body and brain and how those two elements are working together is still a tricky question. Before discussing the practical applications of the serious games, let's have a quick overview of the integration of body and brain.

5.1.1 History and Philosophy

For thousands of years, questions about the soul, mind, and body have been discussed by philosophers, scientists, and doctors. Two major currents have emerged: the dualism, a strict separation between body and soul, developed by Plato, and the monism, considering the body as an indivisible whole, on the other hand. Today, majority of the questions about consciousness remain unanswered.

In medicine and revalidation, it is clear that the dualistic approach still prevails today. Indeed, only a few specialties are interested in the body as a whole and, a fortiori, analyze the links and relations between these two entities.

The new "transhumanist" and "posthumanist" philosophico-medical currents always pinpoint this body–mind dichotomy by considering the brain as a transmitter of commands that can be artificially recreated (neural stimulation, transcranial magnetic stimulation, etc.) and as a hard disk for memories and emotions. Researchers

© Springer International Publishing AG 2018
B. Bonnechère, *Serious Games in Physical Rehabilitation*,
https://doi.org/10.1007/978-3-319-66122-3_5

even focus on "mind uploading," literally downloading the mind and knowledge to a computer. Some scientists believe that fiction will become reality around 2045 (Wiley 2014)!

Yet, as we will see, patients would benefit from a holistic approach by making the most of each entity.

5.1.2   Current Knowledge

A better understanding of mind–body interactions has been made possible by a better understanding of brain's physiology and functioning. Two technologies have allowed major advances in this field, on the one hand, functional imaging of the brain and, on the other hand, brain operations performed on awake patients. The work and the discoveries made in these two fields have shown that the hypotheses of Broca developed nearly 150 years ago were not, fully, correct. According to Broca, each cognitive function is located in a specific area of the brain. A lesion located in this area will automatically cause a loss of the function of this area: the famous aphasia of Broca, for example. Research in functional imaging, nuclear magnetic resonance, magnetoencephalography, and especially brain operations in awake patients during which the neurosurgeon specifically tests various areas of the brain, ensuring him that the patient is always able to perform certain tasks (e.g., talking, playing music, performing calculation) showed that the locations described were not as precise as what was commonly described and admitted and especially that the most important element for brain function was not these areas but the connections between the different regions involved in a neural function (Duffeau 2016). In physical rehabilitation and movements training, it is thus not only important to stimulate the motor cortex but also to stimulate all the different zones involved: premotor cortex, motor, cerebellum, basal ganglia—and the connections between those zones but also the areas in charge of the cognitive functions. It is therefore important to maximize the different types of simulation.

5.1.3   Physical Rehabilitation Using the Brain

The interest of the brain–body relationship is not new in medicine. The best-known example of "brain deception" is the "placebo" effect, the suggestion of the treatment leads to physiologic changes induced by the brain that thinks it has been treated (Finniss et al. 2010). This mechanism also works in the opposite direction, when the administration of a treatment without active principles triggers undesirable effects: the "nocebo" effect (Zaccara et al. 2016).

This principle of luring the brain is also found in physical revalidation in the mirror therapy. Created in 1996 and intended initially for amputees of an upper limb, this therapy aims to delude the brain by projecting an image of the limb on the amputated limb, thanks to the use of a mirror (Altschuler et al. 1999). This technique is now applied to hemiplegic patients: the image of the healthy limb is projected of the affected limb. When the patients are moving the healthy limb the brain thinks that it is the affected limb that is moving and significant improvement of the affected limb are observed.

Today, this principle of mirror revalidation is integrated into virtual revalidation solutions: augmented reality (adding visual information that overlays reality) fits perfectly to this theory and allows immersion and more complex motions than those possible with the simple mirror.

We have already seen that virtual reality and new technologies allow to (re)create environment to perform dual-task training. There are many possibilities to perform cognitive tasks coupled with motor activity or to disturb the brain (e.g., inversion of left and right movements, top and bottom) and force it to use and create other neural connection.

In addition to these techniques of virtual reality, simple cognitive exercises carried out using video games would have a favorable effect on the physical condition. We already presented this study that demonstrated the positive effect of a daily program of 12 mental training sessions with the game "How old is your brain" directly after the total hip replacement. After this program, mentally trained patients showed a better clinical outcome than those in the control group while they did not have more physical exercises than in the control group. Mental activity improves the revalidation of patients after total hip replacement (Lehrl et al. 2012). This proves the importance of neuronal plasticity and the complexity of the different neural circuits responsible for motor function.

Another study demonstrated the close interaction between brain and body. Researchers studied the correlation between the activation on the prefrontal cortex during the gait and the risk of fall. They observed that prefrontal brain activity levels while performing a cognitively demanding walking condition predicted falls in high-functioning seniors. These findings implicate neurobiological processes early in the pathogenesis of falls (Verghese et al. 2017)

5.1.4   Effect on Physical Activity on the Brain

We have seen that a cognitive training has a positive influence on the motor aspects, is the opposite true? Since the 1990s, the number of published studies on the link between physical activity and cognitive performance has increased exponentially. Two questions could be raised: Does physical activity have an immediate and/or long-term effect on cognitive functions?

Concerning the short-term effect, the activation of the cerebral cortex after a period of 20 min of walk compared to a group of subjects that do not move is much more important, leading de facto to an increase in cognitive abilities (Hillman et al. 2009).

For the long-term effect, a meta-analysis published in Nature summarized the different researches performed: a positive correlation between aerobic capacities and computing and reading capacities has been demonstrated (Hillman et al. 2008).

The type of exercise (endurance, explosive effort, or strength training) does not seem to influence cognitive performance (Harveson et al. 2016). The choice can therefore be left to the patient according to his abilities and envy.

5.2   Integration of Serious Games in the Conventional Rehabilitation

In the previous chapter, a lot of studies have been presented about the use of serious games to perform physical rehabilitation and the effect of this new approach on several outcomes.

Several approaches are possible to integrate serious games within the rehabilitation. Before discussing those modalities, it is important to discuss a bit about the acceptance of new technology by the physiotherapist and the medical world in general.

From the earliest times, physiotherapy and rehabilitation have been characterized by this special relationship that is established and built up throughout the treatment between the clinician and the patient. This relationship is built on the duration of treatment.

We have seen in the previous chapters the importance of developing new equipment for patients and clinicians. This technological development, coupled with the evolution of computers and related disciplines: Big Data, Data Mining, Artificial Intelligence, offers, and will offer, every day new possibilities and perspectives in the fields of rehabilitation and medicine.

It is therefore no longer a question of whether technology and informatics will be developed and used in the field of healthcare or not but a question of time. The technophobic and retrograde attitude of some people would not allow a constructive debate and an enlightened and enlightening vision.

It is interesting to note that misoneism, which aims at rejecting any innovation, is not specific to technology or healthcare. There are plenty of examples in the literature of these neophobes: scientists, philosophers, professors, etc.

Several scenarios are possible to accept the technology or not and the computer in health care system from the most conservative: total rejection of the use of technology to the most technophile one that would like to replace human by robots and computers. We will discuss this question in the next chapter.

From now on let's consider that the technology is a support and a help for both clinicians and patients and let's see how to use it and integrate it in different phases of the rehabilitation process.

5.2.1 Early Phase

Patients with some pathologies, such as acute stroke, polytrauma, and severe burns, could not move during the early stages of management and hospitalization. Currently, the treatment during this phase is mainly focusing on the prevention of associated complications (e.g., bedsores, thrombosis).

We have just seen that brain training could have a positive influence on the body and on motor performance; therefore, it could be interesting to try to use those connections and interactions in the very early phase of the management of such complex pathologies.

Two possibilities could be considered (in the context of this book):

The first one is the use of mental training and brain imagery to (r)establish synaptic connection and create new neural networks that will later help with the physical rehabilitation process. Serious games can be used in this phase to help the patients to think about the motion they need to perform. Actually in this part, this is not really games but movies of the games, when the patient is seeing the avatar performing some motions and tasks in the games he is integrating the information in the area of the brain involved in the programmation of the motion. Many affordables and easy-to-use electroencephalography devices (approximately 400€) are currently being developed with a relatively small amount of sensors (16–20). The spatial accuracy is thus limited, and it is difficult to link electroencephalography activities to motion (e.g., the studies trying to use EEG signals to control prosthesis are not advanced enough yet). So such kind of devices is not ready yet but with the exponential development of technologies and artificial intelligence it should be possible in a few years.

The second one is the use of surface electromyography. This is obviously possible only when patients are still able to control and contract the muscles but electrical activity can be detected and recorded even if the patients are not moving. Once again thanks to the development of affordable (350€) wireless and easy-to-use electromyography devices, researchers and developers try to integrate those devices within some rehabilitation exercises (Liu et al. 2016). This method presents lots of advantages: rehabilitation can really start in the early phase of the medical care, patients have to learn to contract one specific muscle (or group of muscles) in order to avoid co-contraction (co-contraction is a frequent consequence of neurologic disease that causes difficulties in gross and fine motor control); although there is no motion, the different systems involved in motor generation and control could be preserved and finally it could speed up the brain plasticity.

Currently, this is only hypothetical and based on previous studies and theories there is no trial supporting such kind of intervention yet because it is only being developed now.

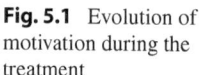 **Fig. 5.1** Evolution of motivation during the treatment

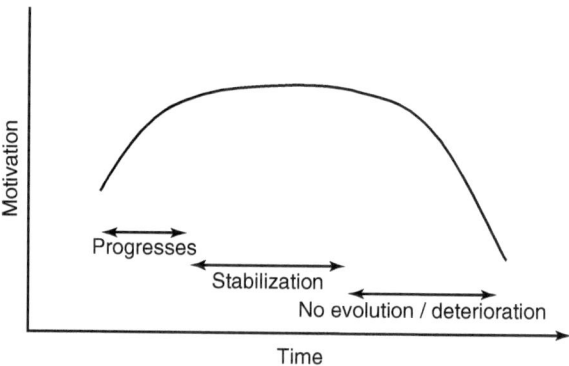

5.2.2   During the Treatment

All the studies about the integration of serious games within the conventional rehabilitation process are currently being performed during the treatment.

Results of different studies (RCTs, cohorts, case studies) have been presented in the previous chapter. There is an important aspect that needs to be taken into consideration: the translational aspect of the research. To say it simply, it is the way to integrate research (fundamental and applied) directly to the patient in clinics. Some studies have shown great results in the very strict and controlled environment of RCT for a new drug, medical devices, or rehabilitation techniques (efficacy) but when the treatment is applied in daily clinics the results are not as good as expected during the research and validation process (effectiveness).

Same problems could occur with the serious games. Of course, serious games must be based on clinical schemes, be motivating for the patients even for a long period and easy to use for both clinicians and patients. Maybe the most important point is to decide when and how to integrate the games in the treatment: based on the motivation or based on the amount of exercises.

We already discussed and highlighted the importance of motivation during the rehabilitation. Figure 5.1 shows the typical evolution of the motivation of the patient during the rehabilitation: during the first sessions, the patients are motivated and they progress, then there is a plateau the evolution is slower and then finally there is a lack of motivation when there is no more progress or when there is deterioration of the status, the exercises are always the same. Therefore integrating the serious games during this period before the fall of motivation is a good option considering the motivational point of view. Most of the patients like novelty and this will boost them and encourage them to continue the rehabilitation.

Another approach is to consider the amount of exercises and motions that the patients are doing. In the beginning of the treatment, the sessions are close to one another and the patients do not need to do that much exercises without the physiotherapist. Then, progressively the sessions are getting more and more spaced and the patients are asked to perform at-home exercises. Unfortunately, it is known that only 30% of the patients did all the prescribed exercises at home (Bonnechère et al.

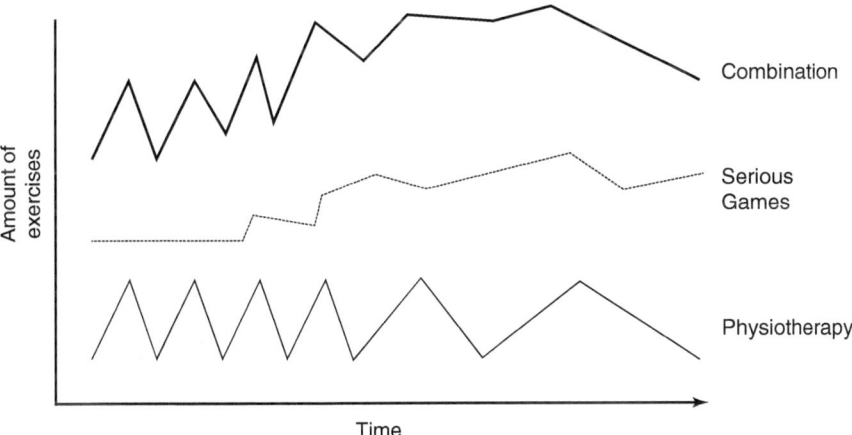

Fig. 5.2 Example of "cooperative" work between conventional physiotherapy and serious games

2016). In order to maintain a high amount of exercises, the serious games can be integrated progressively first during the rehabilitation session with the help and supervision of the physiotherapist and then being progressively installed at home to help the patients form a motivational point of view (Fig. 5.2). The games can also be used to correct the exercises and provide feedback for both patients and clinicians (see Chap. 7 about the future developments) (Fig. 5.2).

5.2.3   After the Treatment

Too often after the rehabilitation, patients do not perform any exercises anymore. This could be potentially problematic since a lot of these exercises are more preventive than curative. Patient empowerment has been highlighted and is encouraged by lot of national health system and professionals. It has been proved that it induces a reduction of the cost related to healthcare and treatment. Another interesting point is that there is a decreased the risk of relapse when the patients are more active in the treatment.

In order to turn the patient from a passive situation to an active one, the information is very important and after the treatment the possibilities offered by the serious games should definitely not be neglected from the motivational point of view but it can act as a reminder for the patients to perform some exercises. Furthermore, there is very often visualization tools, in the specific system not in the commercial video games, that allows a follow-up of the progress done by the patients that could stimulate them.

References

Altschuler EL, Wisdom SB, Stone L, Foster C, Galasko D, Llewellyn DM, Ramachandran VS. Rehabilitation of hemiparesis after stroke with a mirror. Lancet. 1999;353(9169):2035–6.

Bonnechère B, Jansen B, Omelina L, Van Sint Jan S. Do patients perform their exercises at home and why (not)? A survey on patients' habits during rehabilitation exercises. Ulutas Med J. 2016;2(1):41–6.

Duffeau H. L'erreur de Broca. Paris, France: Michel Lafon; 2016.

Finniss DG, Kaptchuk TJ, Miller F, Benedetti F. Biological, clinical, and ethical advances of placebo effects. Lancet. 2010;375(9715):686–95.

Harveson AT, Hannon JC, Brusseau TA, Podlog L, Papadopoulos C, Durrant LH, Hall MS, Kang KD. Acute effects of 30 minutes resistance and aerobic exercise on cognition in a high school sample. Res Q Exerc Sport. 2016;9:1–7.

Hillman CH, Erickson KI, Kramer AF. Be smart, exercise your heart: exercise effects on brain and cognition. Nat Rev Neurosci. 2008;9(1):58–65. Review

Hillman CH, Pontifex MB, Raine LB, Castelli DM, Hall EE, Kramer AF. The effect of acute treadmill walking on cognitive control and academic achievement in preadolescent children. Neuroscience. 2009;159(3):1044–54.

Lehrl S, Gusinde J, Schulz-Drost S, Rein A, Schlechtweg PM, Jacob H, Krinner S, Gelse K, Pauser J, Brem MH. Advancement of physical process by mental activation: a prospective controlled study. J Rchabil Res Dev. 2012;49(8):1221–8.

Liu L, Chen X, Lu Z, Cao S, Wu, Zhang X. Development of an EMG-ACC-based upper limb rehabilitation training system. IEEE Trans Neural Syst Rehabil Eng. 2016.; [Epub ahead of print]

Verghese J, Wang C, Ayers E, Izzetoglu M, Holtzer R. Brain activation in high-functioning older adults and falls: prospective cohort study. Neurology. 2017;88(2):191–7.

Wiley K. A taxonomy and metaphysics of mind-uploading. Los Angeles: Humanity+ Press/ Alautun Press; 2014.

Zaccara G, Giovannelli F, Giorgi FS, Franco V, Gasparini S. Analysis of nocebo effects of antiepileptic drugs across different conditions. J Neurol. 2016;263(7):1274–9.

The Need of Clinical Validation

6

> *Ultimately, I feel that will be a key to the success of this watch,*
> *or any new wearable technology. With validation will come*
> *utilization and ultimately success.*
>
> – *Jon Meyer*

6.1 Introduction

One of the conclusions of this review was that there was a lack of standardization for protocol (e.g., duration and number of sessions) and outcome measurements. Therefore, it is difficult to compare the studies published in this domain. However, there is sufficient evidence in support of SG to allow its inclusion in conventional treatment.

In this chapter, we are going to present a protocol designed for the validation of the integration of serious games in the treatment of children with cerebral palsy (CP) (e.g. Sharan et al. 2012). The protocol, (e.g. number of patients, tests used) can be adapted for other pathologies, the number of patients and the tests used must be adapted.

To increase levels of evidence, it is important to adopt standardized protocols (i.e., interventions, populations, and outcomes) and use common tools, allowing comparison between studies (Van Sint Jan et al. 2015). The aim of this large, multicenter study is to present a protocol to validate the use of SGs in conventional physical rehabilitation treatment for children with CP, using specially developed solutions.

© Springer International Publishing AG 2018
B. Bonnechère, *Serious Games in Physical Rehabilitation*,
https://doi.org/10.1007/978-3-319-66122-3_6

6.2   Designs of RCTs to Validate the use of Serious Games

6.2.1   Design

The study will be a multicenter interventional randomized controlled trial (RCT). It will be a single-blind experiment: all testing will be performed by clinicians who are unaware of the group allocation. Because of the nature of the intervention, it is not possible to perform a double- or triple-blind study.

6.2.2   Setting

The flow chart for patient selection and repartition is presented in Fig. 6.1. The duration of the intervention will be 3 months. The patients will be randomly allocated to one of three groups:

- One group receiving standard physiotherapy
- One group receiving standard physiotherapy (50%) combined with SGs (50%)
- One group receiving only SGs

The intervention involving SGs is described in Sects. 6.2.4 and 6.2.5 below.

Five different evaluations will be performed during the study: one before the intervention (baseline); two during the intervention (one per month), to determine the best duration for the intervention; one immediately after the intervention; and

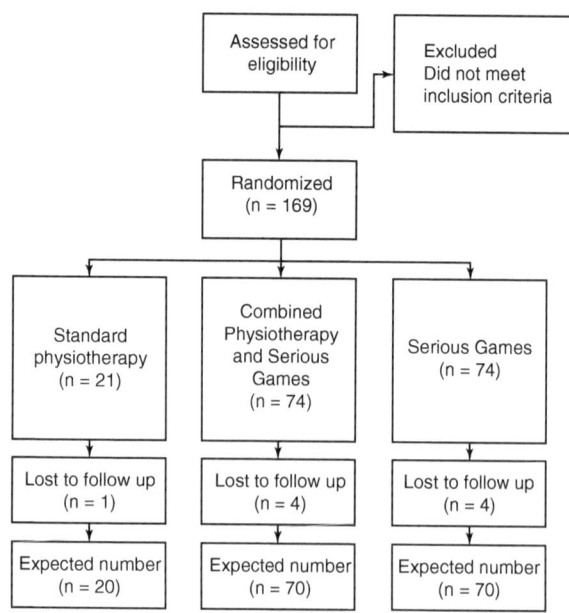

Fig. 6.1 Flow chart for the study and patient selection

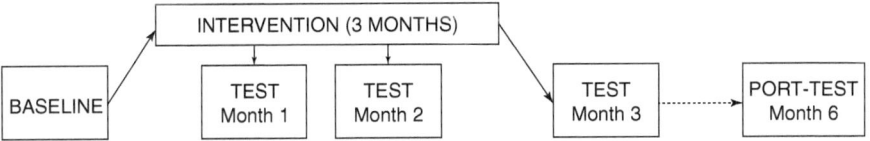

Fig. 6.2 Timeline for the study, with the intervention steps and evaluations in the protocol

one 3 months after the intervention, to determine whether progress is maintained over time (the timeline for the study is presented in Fig. 6.2).

6.2.3   Participants

The inclusion criteria will include the age 6–18 years, a diagnosis of CP, the ability to stand (Gross Motor Function Classification System [GMFCS]: I-II-III), and the ability to understand the instructions (no cognitive [minimum IQ: >70] or language problems). The exclusion criteria will include use of trunk support, behavioral disorders, orthopedic interventions or botulinum toxin injections in the preceding 6 months, and the use of an intrathecal baclofen pump.

6.2.4   Materials

A platform for physical rehabilitation for children with CP, which includes specially developed serious games, has been designed and validated (Omelina et al. 2012). Several mini-games are available. Screenshots, descriptions of the games, and the therapeutic objectives of each game are presented in Tables 6.1 and 6.2. The system included a powerful configuration interface that allows the clinician to set all of the game (e.g., speed, visual complexity, and sounds) and play (e.g., joints and required range of motion) parameters. Therefore, each set of games can be adapted according to patient need and specificity (Omelina et al. 2012). Screenshots and explanations for this configuration interface are presented in Fig. 6.3. A Kinect™ sensor is used to control the games involving limb and trunk displacement, and a Wii Balance Board™ (WBB) is used for balance and posture training. This system has already been used in a feasibility study involving 10 children with CP (Bonnechère et al. 2017).

6.2.5   Interventions

The duration of the intervention will be 3 months, with three sessions per week, each lasting 30 min. The duration of the intervention and number of sessions are highly dependent on the study, and there is no consensus regarding the best treatment duration or number of sessions in the literature (Bonnechère et al. 2014).

Table 6.1 Descriptions of the specially developed games used in the study

Games		Description	Therapeutic objectives
Pirates		The patient must bring the pirate to the treasure by following the path. The width of the path can be configured. The formation of the path (e.g., lines, curves, and asymmetry) can be modified to increase difficulty	Fine adjustment of joint control to keep the pirate in line with the treasure. Limb coordination when the game is played using both limbs simultaneously. Visualization of the displacement of the pirates linked to limbs or trunk motion
Wipe out		The aim of the game is to clean the screen, which is covered in mud. The screen can be cleared with one or both hands (in this case, the screen is virtually divided to force the patient to move both limbs). The pictures behind the mud are changed each time, and the physiotherapist can ask questions about the pictures during the exercises	The precision and amplitude required to succeed can be altered according to the sensitivity of the game (see Fig. 6.3 for game configuration). The game requires coordination between the limbs. Visual feedback regarding the zone cleaned with one arm, relative to the other, provides interesting information for patients, particularly those with asymmetric symptoms. Patients are required to raise their arms to clean the upper corners. Repetitions of this type of exercise increase upper limb strength

	Description	Features
Flight simulator	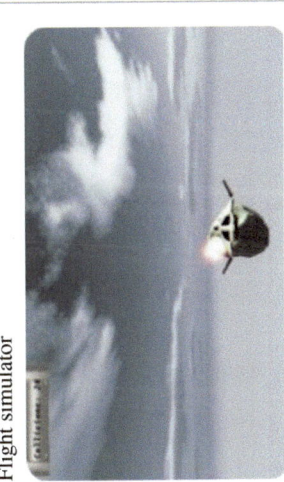 The patient is required to control the plane to collect stars and avoid asteroids. The direction of the plane is limited to medio-lateral displacement (1 direction)	– Control of trunk bending. The plane is controlled via bending; the trunk must remain in the frontal plane – The game can be controlled using the Wii Balance Board™. In this case, the plane is controlled via displacement of the center of pressure – Proprioception can be increased via live visual feedback regarding the plane's movement via displacement of the center of pressure (Balance Board) or the trunk
Hit the box	The aim is to drop the boxes. The patient is required to keep the target in the correct position. After a predefined period (defined in the configuration), the ball is thrown. The direction of the plane is limited to medio-lateral displacement (1 direction)	– Fine adjustment of joint control to keep the target in the correct position – This game can be controlled via the Wii Balance Board™. In this case, the target is controlled via lateral displacement of the center of pressure – This game was developed to increase postural control. Indeed, posture needs to be maintained for a certain period (to be determined by the clinician) before the ball can be thrown – Visualization of displacement of the target linked to joint motion

(continued)

Table 6.1 (continued)

Games		Description	Therapeutic objectives
Drop the ball		The patient is required to control the ball to ensure that it falls into the correct basket, by controlling the two boards. According to the therapeutic objectives of the game, the plates are controlled via the arms, trunk, or displacement of the center of pressure	– This game requires displacement of the center of pressure (in cases involving use of the Wii Balance Board™) or coordination between the arms (to control the upper plate) or the upper limbs and trunk (in cases involving use of the Kinect™ alone) to control the lower plate – The lower plate can be controlled via the Wii Balance Board™. In this case, the inclination of the plate is controlled via lateral displacement of the center of pressure – Visualization of displacement of the plates linked to arm motion and displacement of the center of pressure – Players are required to keep their arms flexed (approximately 90° of flexion) during the entire game. This task requires isometric contraction of the brachialis and deltoids (anterior head)
Mushrooms		The aim is to collect as many mushrooms as possible. The game was developed for hemiplegic patients with limbs in "triple flexion." The game forces patients to stretch out the affected limb to collect the mushrooms. It also requires the control of trunk bending (to orient towards the other mushrooms in the environment). The game increases coordination between affected and unaffected limbs	– It is necessary for patients to control the position of the trunk (lateral bending) to collect the mushrooms. The trunk has to remain in a vertical position during the collection of the mushrooms and bend to rotate the environment – Two body segments are targeted. Proprioception of the trunk: the trunk must remain motionless, otherwise the environment will rotate. Proprioception of the limbs (particularly the affected one): he limb must be stretched outwards to collect mushrooms in a 3D environment

Table 6.2 Summary of the therapeutic objectives of each game
Dark green **main target,** *light green* **secondary target,** *red* **not targeted**

Game	Motor Control	Balance	Posture	Proprioception	Strengthening
Wipeout	dark green	red	light green	light green	dark green
Mushrooms	dark green	red	red	light green	red
Flight simulator	light green	dark green	red	light green	red
Hit the box	light green	dark green	dark green	dark green	red
The pirates	light green	red	red	light green	red
Drop the ball	dark green	dark green	red	dark green	dark green

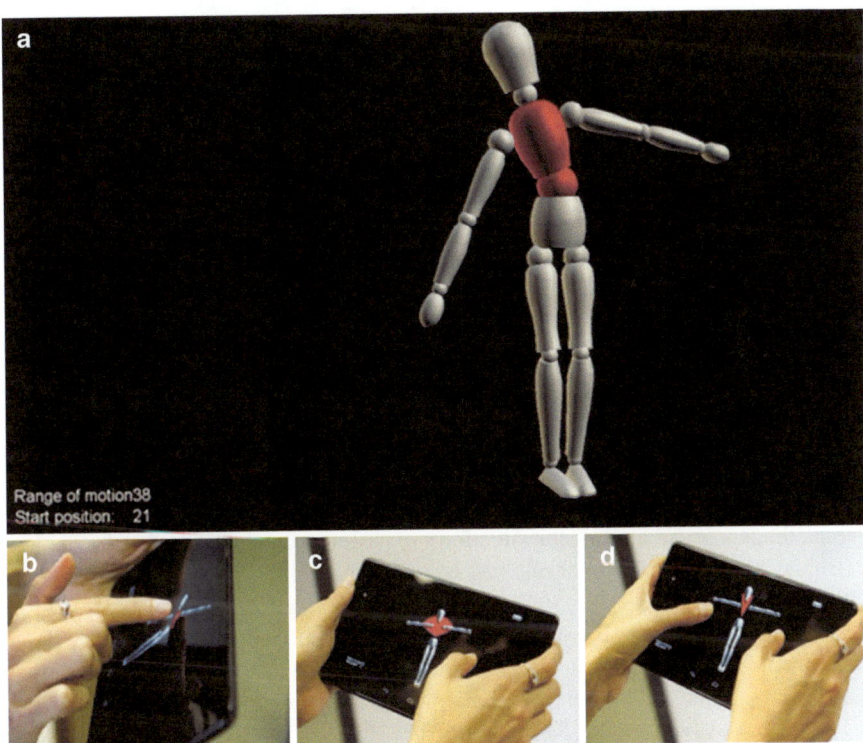

Range of motion 38
Start position: 21

Fig. 6.3 (**a**) Configuration interface used to adapt the games to each patient. (**b**) A single touch is used to select a body segment. (**c**) An up-down gesture is used to specify the neutral position for the selected body segment. (**d**) A gesture involving two fingers is used to specify the range of motion for the selected joint

Therefore, we will perform intermediate evaluations during the intervention to analyze the patients' progress (if any) over time and define the best duration for the intervention in future clinical use.

For the group receiving SG exercises, the order of the games and configuration used (game controllers and joints involved) will be defined at random to avoid effects of habituation or fatigue. Each game will be played for 5 min (3 different games in the group receiving combined physiotherapy and SGs, and 6 in the group receiving only SGs). At the end of the intervention, each game will be played for the same amount of time.

Relative to commercial video games, one of the advantages of specific games in rehabilitation is that they can be configured and adapted according to patient need and specificity. The games will be configured by a trained therapist during the first session of the intervention. This configuration will be modified according to the patients' progress (or a familiarization with the games) after 1 and 2 months, to ensure that it is suits their abilities.

With respect to the standard physiotherapy, the therapist will not receive particular instructions, with the exception of those regarding the duration of the session, which is fixed to 30 min for the group receiving standard physiotherapy alone and 15 min for the group receiving standard physiotherapy combined with 15 min of SGs.

6.2.6 Outcomes

Several parameters will be evaluated during the study. A distinction will be made between the tests performed during evaluations (Fig. 6.2) and continuous follow-up performed during rehabilitation exercises.

6.2.7 Evaluation

All of the tests that will be performed during the five evaluations are presented in Table 6.3.

Balance and posture: Two different approaches are available to assess balance (e.g., diagnosis and treatment evaluation): quantitative evaluation using force plates (Bonnechère et al. 2015b) or qualitative evaluation using a clinical scale (Heyrman et al. 2011).

Qualitative balance assessments will be performed using the qualitative Trunk Control Measurement Scale (Heyrman et al. 2011), which is subdivided into three categories: static sitting balance, dynamic sitting balance, and dynamic reaching. The total possible score is 58 points for healthy subjects (i.e., 20 points for static sitting, 28 points for dynamic sitting, and 10 points for dynamic reaching). The scale has previously been used to evaluate trunk control before and after an SG intervention (Bonnechère et al. 2017).

Quantitative balance assessments will be performed using the WBB coupled to software to obtain parameters derived from center of pressure (CoP) displacement

Table 6.3 Tests used to assess patients

Test		Baseline	Intervention			Post-test
		1	2	3	4	5
TCMS	Static sitting (/20)					
	Dynamic sitting (/28)					
	Dynamic reaching (/10)					
	Total (58)					
Balance	Bipedal—eyes open					
	Right leg—eyes open					
	Left leg—eyes open					
	Bipedal—eyes closed					
	Right leg—eyes closed					
	Left leg—eyes closed					
FMS	Home (/6)					
	School (/6)					
	Community (/6)					
	Total (/18)					
PEDI	Self-care (/73)					
	Mobility (/59)					
	Social function (/65)					
	Total (/197)					
MUUL (/122)						
PedsQL	Physical health (/100)					
	Psychosocial health (/100)					
	Total (/100)					
SFQ-child						
Borg scale of perceived exertion (/20)						

FMS functional mobility scale, *MUUL* Melbourne assessment of unilateral upper limb function, *PEDI* pediatric evaluation of disability inventory, *PedsQL* pediatric quality of life inventory, *SFQ* short feedback questionnaire, *TCMS* trunk control measurement scale

(Bonnechère et al. 2015b). Patients will be asked to stand on the WBB for 30 s. Different conditions will be tested: bipedal and unipedal with eyes open and closed. The parameters derived from CoP will include total displacement of sway, the area of the 95% prediction ellipse (often referred to as the 95% confidence ellipse); dispersion of CoP displacement from the mean position, the distance between maximum and minimum CoP displacement, mean velocity for CoP displacement; and anterior-posterior and medio-lateral displacement of the total CoP sway divided by the total duration of the trial (total mean velocity). We decided to use the WBB instead of a laboratory force plate to facilitate the organization of the study. All of the experiments can be conducted in the institutions, and patients will not need to visit a gait laboratory. Several studies have validated the use of the WBB to assess balance and posture in patients with neurological diseases in clinical contexts (e.g., multiple sclerosis (Castelli et al. 2015) and Parkinson's disease (Holmes et al. 2013)).

Gross motor function: The Functional Mobility Scale, which is completed by parents and measures children's ability to move in various situations (e.g., at home and at school) will be used to assess gross motor function (Harvey et al. 2010). The Pediatric Evaluation of Disability Inventory will be used to evaluate patients' autonomy, mobility, and social function (Dumas et al. 2010). The GMFCS and the Manual Ability Classification System (Compagnone et al. 2014) will be used to define the population during the first evaluation.

Fine motor control in the upper limbs: The Melbourne Assessment of Unilateral Upper Limb Function (MUUL), which is an objective tool that evaluates upper limb function in children with CP, will be used to assess upper limb function. Several functions, such as grasping, releasing, and object manipulation, will be assessed.

Quality of life: Quality of life will be assessed using the Pediatric Quality of Life Inventory (PedsQL). The PedsQL is a brief, standardized, generic assessment instrument that systematically evaluates patients' and parents' perceptions of health-related quality of life in pediatric patients with chronic health conditions (Varni et al. 1999).

Patient's satisfaction: The Short Feedback Questionnaire for Children will be used to assess patients' responses while performing exercises. This scale evaluates 8 items: enjoyment, sense of presence, success, control, perception of the environment as realistic, the understandability of feedback from the games, discomfort, and difficulty level (Weiss et al. 2004). The Borg Scale of Perceived Exertion will be used to assess patients' perceived physical effort, with responses provided using a scale ranging from 6 (no exertion) to 20 (maximum exertion possible) (Borg 1990).

6.2.8   Continuous Follow-Up

All of the motions performed by the patients will be recorded via the game controllers (Kinect™ and WBB). Dynamic evaluation of the balance will be performed for the games played using the WBB. The same parameters as those used for the quantitative balance assessment will be used to perform this follow-up. Depending on the games and configurations used, different scores will be derived from the games played using the Kinect™ (Bonnechère et al. 2015a; Sholukha et al. 2015).

6.2.9   Statistical Analysis

The normality of the data will be assessed using Kolmogorov-Smirnov tests. ANOVAs will be performed to compare results of the five evaluations. In cases involving difference, post hoc tests will be performed using the Bonferroni procedure. To identify the patients who benefit most from the intervention, progress made between baseline and the mid-term intervention (assessment at 2 months) will be evaluated and expressed in percentages using Eq. (6.1), before examining correlations between this score and GMFCS and Manual Ability Classification System classification.

$$\text{Normalized difference} = \frac{\text{Post-intervention test} - \text{Pre-intervention test}}{\text{Pre-intervention test}} \times 100 \quad (6.1)$$

The same procedure will be applied before the baseline and final (3 months after the intervention) evaluations to determine whether there is a correlation between the progress made during the intervention, assessed immediately after the intervention, and retention.

The characteristics of the tests used to assess the patients were used to estimate the required sample size. We set the expected differences for the tests just above the standard error of measurement for each test. Because of the heterogeneity of the sample size estimation, we chose the highest value (for the MUUL and PedsQL) and set the sample size at 70. Based on this value, we calculated power and obtained a mean β of 0.86 for all tests (lowest β was that of the MUUL [0.77]).

6.3   Discussion

Because of the complexity of CP, management is a complex task that requires the involvement of a multidisciplinary team. Rehabilitation exercises must be performed as frequently as possible to avoid spasticity and related consequences (e.g., vicious attitudes or bone deformation). These exercises (at home or with a physiotherapist) are subject to several problems. The first involves a lack of patient motivation, with only 30% of patients performing the exercises regularly at home (Sluijs et al. 1993). The second is that exercises performed at home are not supervised by a clinician, and there is no feedback provided for either patients or therapists. The third involves difficulties in gaining access to care, which are roughly categorized as either financial or physical. For these physically impaired children and their caregivers, the need to travel to a rehabilitation center frequently is a serious burden. The World Health Organization highlighted lack of access to available rehabilitation services, particularly in low-income countries and rural areas, as a major barrier to rehabilitation (WHO 2011). All of these problems could be solved by the use of SGs in rehabilitation. For example, the development of rehabilitation schemes based on SGs could compensate for the lack of therapists in some emerging countries. A pilot-study pertaining to this topic was conducted in Jamaica (Gordon et al. 2012), and SGs could be used to provide feedback for patients and ensure that they are performing the exercises correctly (Bonnechère et al. 2013).

Despite these benefits, the important question as to the efficacy of SGs when used for children with CP remains unanswered (Bonnechère et al. 2014). The lack of evidence in this regard could result from the protocol used. Indeed, in most previous studies, SGs are added to conventional therapy; therefore, it is impossible to determine whether the observed outcomes result from the use of SG or an increase in rehabilitation time. For this reason, the proposed study will involve three branches: one involving conventional physical therapy, one involving a combination of conventional therapy and SGs, and one involving SGs alone. From an ethical perspective, some would argue that it is unacceptable to deprive children with CP of their regular therapy in favor of a new treatment for which there is no supportive evidence. However, several points address this concern. First, conventional therapy will not be lost to these children indefinitely; they will receive a different type of

Table 6.4 Sample size estimation and power analyses

Test	Mean (SD)	SEM	Expected difference	N	β (n = 70)
TCMS (Heyrman et al. 2011)	38 (8)	2	3	44	0.93
Balance (Clark et al. 2010)	48 (13)	5	6	30	0.99
PEDI (Berg et al. 2004)	143 (35)	10	11	63	0.84
MUUL (Klingels et al. 2008)	57 (14)	3	4	69	0.77
PedsQL (Tantilipikorn et al. 2013)	71 (17)	4	5	72	0.79

Power analyses were performed based on 70 patients

MUUL Melbourne assessment of unilateral upper limb function, *PEDI* pediatric evaluation of disability inventory, *PedsQL* pediatric quality of life inventory, *SD* standard deviation, *SEM* standard error of measurement, *TCMS* trunk control measurement scale

therapy for 3 months before returning to their original rehabilitation. Second, there are good indications from pilot studies (Bonnechère et al. 2017) and previous research that children who receive therapy involving SGs are not worse than children who receive regular therapy. The management and treatment of CP in children is a complex, multidisciplinary, multidimensional task with numerous parameters that require consideration. The complexity and heterogeneity of the clinical presentation of CP make it difficult to obtain scientific evidence for treatments and interventions. Therefore, most of the treatments currently used in daily practice for children with CP are not based on scientific evidence (Bonnechère et al. 2014).

Another weakness in previous studies was the sample size. Because of the nature of the pathology and heterogeneity of the symptomatology, it is difficult to perform large-scale studies; however, depending on the characteristics of tests and pathology (see Sect. 6.2.9 and Table 6.4), a large number of patients are likely to be required to demonstrate clinically significant differences. In this particular context, a multi-center trial is required to facilitate patient recruitment and inclusion. Another advantage of conducting multicenter trials is that they are less dependent on the enthusiasm of one particular clinician (e.g., the researcher), and feedback and information can be obtained from different specialists. This approach is closer to clinical application relative to monocenter trials performed by one therapist.

One last point that requires discussion is that of game choice. We have discussed the difference between commercial and specially developed games above. The advantages of specific games adapted for rehabilitation are somewhat obvious. Of course, this type of research could be conducted with numerous different games for the target group. However, we have chosen to frame it in the context of a specific set of games that have been developed in close collaboration with clinicians (e.g., medical doctors, physiotherapists, and occupational therapists), patients, and their relatives.

References

Berg M, Jahnsen R, Frøslie KF, Hussain A. Reliability of the pediatric evaluation of disability inventory (PEDI). Phys Occup Ther Pediatr. 2004;24(3):61–77.

Bonnechère B, Jansen B, Omelina L, Da Silva L, Mouraux D, Rooze M, Van Sint Jan S. Patient follow-up using serious games. A feasibility study on low back pain patients. In: Schouten B, Fedtke S, Bekker T, Schijven M, Gekker A, editors. Games for health. Wiesbaden: Springer; 2013. p. 185–95.

Bonnechère B, Jansen B, Omelina L, Degelaen M, Wermenbol V, Rooze M, Van Sint Jan S. Can serious games be incorporated with conventional treatment of children with cerebral palsy? A review. Res Dev Disabil. 2014;35(8):1899–913.

Bonnechère B, Jansen B, Omelina L, Diaz F, Sholukha V, Van Sint Jan S. Clinical evolution of familiarization? Time analysis of serious games exercises to assess the learning effect. In: ICVR Congress, Valencia, Spain, 2015a.

Bonnechère B, Jansen B, Omelina L, Van Sint Jan S. Interchangeability of the Wii Blanace board™ for bipedal balance assessment. JMIR Rehabilitation and Assistive Technologies. 2015b;2(2):e8.

Bonnechère B, Omelina L, Jansen B, Van Sint Jan S. Balance improvement after physical therapy training using specially developed serious games for cerebral palsy children: preliminary results. Disabil Rehabil. 2017;39(4):403–6.

Borg G. Psychophysical scaling with applications in physical work and the perception of exertion. Scand J Work Environ Health. 1990;16(S1):55–8.

Castelli L, Stocchi L, Patrignani M, Sellitto G, Giuliani M, Prosperini L. We-measure: toward a low-cost portable posturography for patients with multiple sclerosis using the commercial Wii balance board. J Neurol Sci. 2015;359(1-2):440–4.

Clark RA, Bryant AL, Pua Y, McCrory P, Bennell K, Hunt M. Validity and reliability of the Nintendo Wii balance board for assessment of standing balance. Gait Posture. 2010 Mar;31(3):307–10.

Compagnone E, Maniglio J, Camposeo S, Vespino T, Losito L, De Rinaldis M, Gennaro L, Trabacca A. Functional classifications for cerebral palsy: correlations between the gross motor function classification system (GMFCS), the manual ability classification system (MACS) and the communication function classification system (CFCS). Res Dev Disabil. 2014;35(11):2651–7.

Dumas H, Fragala-Pinkham M, Haley S, Coster W, Kramer J, Kao YC, Moed R. Item bank development for a revised pediatric evaluation of disability inventory (PEDI). Phys Occup Ther Pediatr. 2010;30:168–84.

Gordon C, Roopchand-Martin S, Gregg A. Potential of the Nintendo Wii™ as a rehabilitation tool for children with cerebral palsy in a developing country: a pilot study. Physiotherapy. 2012;98(3):238–42.

Harvey AR, Morris ME, Graham HK, Wolfe R, Baker R. Reliability of the functional mobility scale for children with cerebral palsy. Phys Occup Ther Pediatr. 2010;30:139–49.

Heyrman L, Molenaers G, Desloovere K, Verheyden G, De Cat J, Monbaliu E, Feys H. A clinical tool to measure trunk control in children with cerebral palsy: the trunk control measurement scale. Res Dev Disabil. 2011;32(6):2624–35.

Holmes JD, Jenkins ME, Johnson AM, Hunt MA, Clark RA. Validity of the Nintendo Wii® balance board for the assessment of standing balance in Parkinson's disease. Clin Rehabil. 2013;27(4):361–6.

Klingels K, De Cock P, Desloovere K, Huenaerts C, Molenaers G, Van Nuland I, Huysmans A, Feys H. Comparison of the Melbourne assessment of unilateral upper limb function and the quality of upper extremity skills test in hemiplegic CP. Dev Med Child Neurol. 2008;50(12):904–9.

Omelina L., Jansen B., Bonnechère B., Van Sint Jan S., Cornelis J.. 2012. Serious games for physical rehabilitation: designing highly configurable and adaptable games. In: Proceedings of the 9th International Conference on Disability, Virtual Reality & Associated Technologies, Laval, France 195–201.

Sharan D, Ajeesh PS, Rameshkumar R, Mathankumar M, Paulina RJ, Manjula M. Virtual reality based therapy for post operative rehabilitation of children with cerebral palsy. Work. 2012;41(S1):3612–5.

Sholukha V, Bonnechère B, Van Sint Jan S. Trajectory-based analysis, a new method for motion analysis using the Kinect™ sensor. In: ISB 2015, Glasgow, Scotland, 2015.

Sluijs EM, Kok GJ, van der Zee J. Correlates of exercise compliance in physical therapy. Phys Ther. 1993;73(11):771–82. discussion 783-6

Tantilipikorn P, Watter P, Prasertsukdee S. Comparison between utility of the Thai pediatric quality of life inventory 4.0 generic Core scales and 3.0 cerebral palsy module. Int J Rehabil Res. 2013;36(1):21–9.

Van Sint Jan S, Bonnechère B, Moureau D, Brassine E, Sholukha V, Moiseev F. Novel solution for performing regular objective functional assessments for follow-up of neuro-muscular disorders. Physiotherapy. 2015;101(S1):e1577–8.

Varni JW, Seid M, Rode CA. The PedsQL: measurement model for the pediatric quality of life inventory. Med Care. 1999;37(2):126–39.

Weiss PL, Rand D, Katz N, Kizony R. Video capture virtual reality as a flexible and effective rehabilitation tool. J Neuroeng Rehabil. 2004;1(1):12.

World Health Organization (WHO). World Health Organization (WHO) & World Bank world report on disability. Geneva: WHO; 2011.

In the Future 7

The best way to predict your future is to create it.

– Abraham Lincoln

7.1 Problems to Solve

Although the fact that serious games have been tested since several years in clinics, there are still a lot of problems to be solved before using them in daily clinics. Some of these problems concern the technology (precision, price, usability) but the biggest problem seems to be the human mind: how to convince people that playing games is not just fun but can really be helpful in rehabilitation? We saw in the previous chapter that well-conducted clinical studies, large-scale Randomized Clinical Trials, are needed because as presented in the Chap. 4 such kind of studies are still missing. Nonetheless in order to conduct such kind of a study, the clinicians must be convinced of the benefits, safety, and the scientific basis of this new approach.

7.1.1 Technological Issues

A lot of new (gaming) devices and technologies have been presented throughout this book as well as plenty of clinical trials and studies on the use of new kind of technology. Nevertheless, the current technology is, currently, not fully adapted to the clinics and further development and improvement are needed.

7.1.1.1 Accuracy and Precision
These two terms are often misused and confounded although they are used for two totally different things. The accuracy of a measurement system is the degree of closeness of measurements of a quantity to that quantity's true value. The precision

© Springer International Publishing AG 2018   133
B. Bonnechère, *Serious Games in Physical Rehabilitation*,
https://doi.org/10.1007/978-3-319-66122-3_7

of a measurement system, related to reproducibility and repeatability, is the degree to which repeated measurements under unchanged conditions show the same results. Several studies have been performed in order to validate the use of gaming devices to perform some simple biomechanical and functional assessment (see Chap. 1). Paradoxically, the biomechanics community appears to be skeptical about the use of this technology with patients during functional analysis, and often does not consider it as a potential complementary tool to standard equipment (Bonnechère et al. 2016).

It appears that scientists are mainly concerned with the accuracy of instruments in order to accept them as clinical tools.

Yet, most of the daily clinical activities rely more on measurement precision rather than on instrument accuracy to perform patient follow-up. The term precision includes reproducibility (i.e., interobserver measurement) and repeatability (i.e., intraobserver measurement).

Previously published studies on the gaming hardware validation have shown that WBB and Kinect hardware accuracy is lower than gold standards (e.g., Clark et al. 2010, Huurnink et al. 2013 for the WBB; Bonnechère et al. 2013, Cippitelli et al. 2015 for the Kinect); for the WBB, these differences were mainly due to the lack of rigorous calibration of the gaming hardware.

However, gaming hardware showed a similar precision to gold standards (Clark et al. 2010 for the WBB; Bonnechère et al. 2013, 2014a, 2014b for the Kinect). This precision seems to indicate that gaming hardware could be useful for clinical applications in order to monitor patients during follow-up activities. As such, and because of their cost-effectiveness and easiness of use, such hardware could be used for very frequent (e.g., weekly) assessments of patients to, for example, quantify their progresses without the need of sending the patients to specialized centers. The latter centers would still be involved to perform a full and detailed analysis at less frequent intervals (e.g., monthly or bi-annual). As the readers can see, there is a high and obvious complementarity between both systems: on the one hand, accurate and very detailed analysis using high-end equipment, on the other hand, precise and very flexible general assessment using cost-effective transportable and intuitive hardware. The availability of the latter hardware would allow more frequent functional analysis in the practice of private therapists or even at the patient's home.

7.1.1.2 Calibration and Customization

Each patient is unique with specific pathology inducing functional impairment and limitations. Therefore, the games used for the rehabilitation of these patients should also be adapted. This is by definition not the case with commercial games in which it is not possible to modify any relevant parameters.

Specific games have been developed to fulfill, partially, the need of rehabilitation and the capacities of these new kinds of "players."

Two different approaches are currently being used to adapt the games for each patient.

If the games are played under therapist supervision, the clinician can configure the different parameters of the games (range of motion, joints, speed, acceleration, visual background and complexity, sounds, etc.) manually. User-friendly interfaces have been developed to enable real-time modifications in these parameters while the patient is playing in order to have direct feedback of these changes (Omelina et al. 2012).

In the future when the system will be installed in patient's home, in a more systematic way, such kind of calibration and customization will be done automatically based on previous and current patient's performances, thanks to machine learning techniques (Nirme et al. 2011; Perez et al. 2011)

7.1.2 Ethical Issues

Several ethical issues are raised by the development of serious games and telemedicine. The new paradigm of communication between the different actors of rehabilitation is presented in Fig. 7.1. The database, including not only the data storage but also the data analysis and data mining tools, is the key piece of telerehabilitation. As such it is put in the middle of the organigram. Data protection authority and

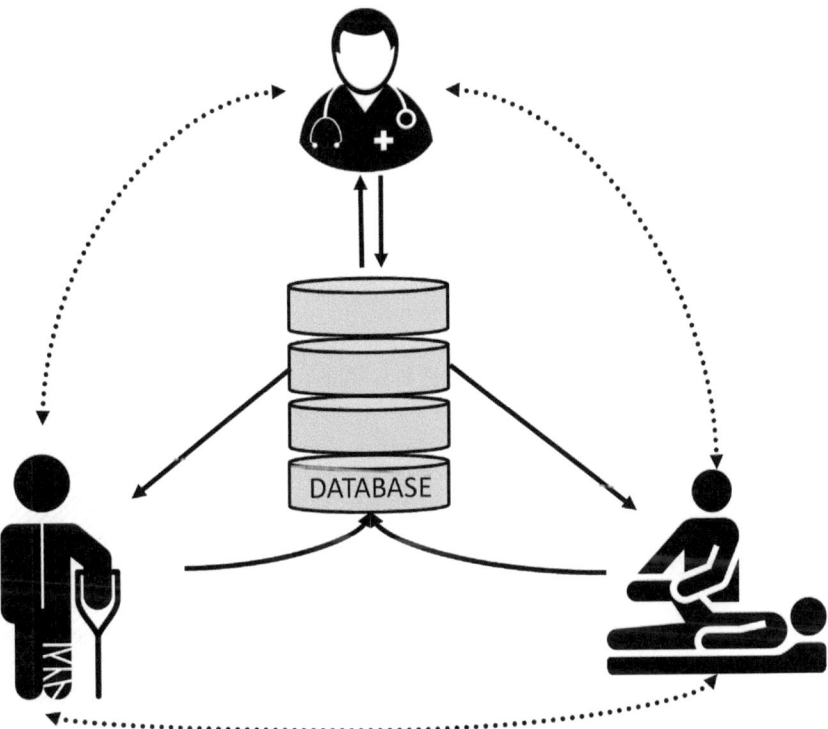

Fig. 7.1 The communication between the different actors of rehabilitation. *Dotted lines* are used to present the traditional and conventional way of communication, *solid lines* are used for telemedicine and telerehabilitation. Note the central position of the database

agencies in charge for the protection of medical data, including ethical committees, pay a lot of attention to the security of databases containing medical or health-related data (encrypted data, patient anonymization). Solid lines represent the communication between patients or clinicians and the database. These connections must also be highly secured and encrypted to allow safe transfer of the health-related data (sensitive data).

Unfortunately, it is almost impossible to guarantee inviolable system since hackers seem able to bypass almost all the security systems, even the more complicated ones. Of course, hackers are more involved in security and financial system but apparently health care services are not spared as illustrated by the case of a hacker having recently taken control of the pacemaker of a patient[1] or hackers tacking control of self-driving cars.

7.1.3   People's Mind

In physical rehabilitation, although there is the world "serious" in it the use of games or serious games is, too often, only associated to fun. Therefore some clinicians, and patients, think that they are only playing and not doing rehabilitation exercises. However, they are doing exactly the same kind of motions in the games that during a conventional rehabilitation session using especially dedicated games.

People are often reluctant to use new technology, especially in the health care sector. The use of games in rehabilitation must thus tackle these two problems: proves that new technologies, issue from the games, and the games themselves can be beneficial in the health care services.

With the "web generation," or the digital native (Prensky 2007), there is no doubt that the mentalities are going to change and there is no reason that these technologies could not be used in rehabilitation; it is certainly just a matter of time.

For the more septic, and more scientific (?), people there is a need of scientific and clinical validation of the use of this new approach in the conventional treatment of different health-related conditions. It is therefore important to conduct clinical validation studies following strict protocol used in clinics to validate new treatment (see Chap. 6).

Ultimately, as final user, patients must be convinced that serious games are beneficial for them. Easy-to-use and user-friendly interfaces must be developed to run the games for all kind of patients (elderly, patients with cognitive impairment, etc.) (Laver et al. 2011). The games must also be easy to play and patients have to understand what they have to do (Plow and Finlayson 2014). Last but not least, the interface must allow a follow-up of the patients and plots the progresses over the time to motivate and stimulate them to perform the rehabilitation exercises during a long time of period.

---

[1] http://www.theatlantic.com/health/archive/2014/11/can-hackers-get-into-your-pacemaker/382893/.

7.1.4   Financial Aspects

We already mentioned the financial issue as potential barrier to rehabilitation. The main and most important question is who is going to pay for this new kind of service. Such kind of device could be installed in private practice, large clinical center (hospital), or at patient's home. Different business model and option must thus be discussed.

In the first case, the material should be bought by the clinician (or group of clinicians), as it is the case with any other health care material. In some cases (choc wave therapy, cryotherapy), clinicians are free to ask a financial participation of the patient in addition to the session.

If the system is installed at home, several scenarios are possible. Either the patient buys the system or he rents it for the duration of the treatment. In this case, is it the clinician who buys the system and rents it to patients (Business-to-Business solution)? Do the companies provide the system with a monthly subscription directly to the patient (Business-to-Customer solution)?

Current companies are relatively young and the products are still in development; therefore, we are not able to provide more information about the best sales strategy or approach.

Last questions: Are the health-care systems going to participate in the reimbursement, fully or partially, of this new kind of intervention? Is it that the patients need to pay everything? What about the use of serious games in emerging countries?

7.2   A Lucrative Market?

7.2.1   Targeted Populations

The benefits generated by the industry of commercial video games are huge: 25 billion dollars estimated for 2014[2]. Compared to this market how important can the serious games industry be? The different pathologies discussed in the Chap. 4 have been listed in Table 7.1. The number of patients suffering from these pathologies in the different region of the world has been estimated.

From a business point of view, three business models are possible: develop products for patients (at-home system), for therapists in private practice (or small center), or for hospital and specialized reference centers (including database for patients follow-up).

From the patient point of view, we have highlighted that the specificity of the treatment is a key point in rehabilitation. It is thus better to use serious games instead of commercial video games because they are adapted to specific pathologies and patients. Therefore, the Table 7.1 should be interpreted line by line rather than by columns because companies must focus on one particular pathology or at least a

---

[2] The Video Gaming Industry Outlook.

Table 7.1 Number of patients suffering from different pathologies in different regions of the world

Pathology	Africa	Americas	Asia	Europe	Oceania	Total (by pathology)
Stroke[a]	2 millions	2.2 millions	19 millions	1.8 millions	100,000	≈ 25 millions
Cerebral palsy	3.3 millions	2.9 millions	13 millions	2.2 millions	120,000	≈ 21.5 millions
Aging (>65 years old)[b]	5.6 millions	138.3 millions (71.6 millions for North America +66.7 millions for Latin America and Caribbean)	476 millions	147 millions	5.8 millions	≈ 770 millions
Obesity	88 millions	262 millions	130 millions	163 millions	2 millions	≈ 645 millions
Parkinson's disease[c]	500,000	1 million	2.15 millions	750,000	50,000	≈ 5 millions
Total (by regions)	99 millions	406 millions	640 millions	315 millions	8 millions	≈1.5 billiards

[a]Number of stroke survivors per year
[b]according to WHO estimation for 2025 (http://www.un.org/esa/population/publications/worldageing19502050/)
[c]Crude prevalence rate

(couple) of clinical signs (e.g., balance, spasticity, coordination) in order to develop specific solutions.

7.2.2 The Current Companies

The aim of this chapter is not to make any kind of advertising for any company; the author is not involved in any of these, but to give an overview of the existing solutions already available for clinicians and patients. This is a non-exhaustive description and all the existing companies are probably not listed here after.

7.2.2.1 Jintronix

This company develops serious games for neurologic rehabilitation using the Kinect sensor.

From a clinician point of view, they claim that the system is useful to improve the quality (clinicians gain access to a range of valid performance metrics and multiple means of displaying improvement) to save time (clinicians don't need to fill in paper since everything is in the system), and to strengthen patients' compliance and motivation.

From the patients point of view, this system is more motivating than traditional at-home rehabilitation exercises, more affordable (patients do not need to go every times to clinicians), and more accessible (clinicians can work remotely).

7.2.2.2 SeeMe Rehabilitation

SeeMe is a computer-based system, innovative and comprehensive solution, offering clinician-controlled exercise and a diagnostic system. It is designed to help the rehabilitation process and track patients' progress. It improves coordination, balance, muscle strength, range of motion, reaction times, and cognitive functions. It also uses Kinect technology.

7.2.2.3 VirtualRehab

According to their creators, VirtualRehab is a clinically validated physical rehabilitation system which uses video games technology and allows the monitoring of the progress of patients from anywhere in the world. The games can be configured according to patients' needs and capabilities.

7.2.2.4 Mira

Mira is a software platform designed to make physiotherapy fun and convenient for patient recovering from surgery or injury. This system transforms existing physical therapy exercises into video games and uses external sensor to track and assess patients' compliance.

7.2.2.5 Rehametrics

Rehametrics, previously Neuro@home, is one solution offering both physical and cognitive rehabilitation within the same product. This solution allows clinicians to prescribe personalized rehabilitation exercises remotely. All the motions performed by the patients are stored and analyzed to get feedback to both patients and therapists. Clinicians can therefore objectively quantify the progress of the patient and adapt the treatment according to the status of the patient.

7.2.2.6 Mitii: Move It to Improve It

Mitii is a solution that combines the newest research of how to prime and boost brain and body and motion tracking using Kinect sensor and tele-technology. Cognitive and physical training are combined in a non-prescriptive way that develops the brains' networks, thus enhancing the foundation on which people learn and increase skills. Mitii is customized to the individual. Training is regularly adjusted in line with the user's progress by the therapist.

7.2.2.7 Valedo

The Valedo's products offer a continuous solution from spine assessment to therapy in the clinic and at home. The Valedo Therapy Concept is developed for patients suffering from low back pain. The system allows clinical assessments and functional exercise training. This company offers both software (the games) and hardware (the device) to perform the rehabilitation exercises and the evaluation.

7.2.2.8 TyroMotion

TyroMotion is a company offering solutions, both software and hardware to perform virtual rehabilitation of various pathologies. Specific materials have been developed to answer relevant clinical questions and requests: balance training, bimanual coordination, robotic system, haptic rehabilitation, etc.

Since their products are developed for rehabilitation, they claim that the evaluation and follow-up is very accurate.

7.3   New Trends

7.3.1   Functional Evaluation During Rehabilitation

We saw in the presentation of the current available commercial products that a lot of solutions allow evaluation and follow-up of the patients. We have also seen that most of these companies are using commercial solution (e.g., Kinect and Balance Board). We already discussed the limits of such kind of hardware (Chap. 1); therefore, novel solutions must be developed (such as Valedo and TyroMotion products) or the available products should be improved.

For example, for the Kinect sensor the skeleton model is composed of only 25 points that are gross estimations of the center of the major joints of the human body. This kind of model only allows simple motion assessment (e.g., vector angle between 3 points for knee or elbow flexion, simple geometric approach to estimate elbow abduction between shoulder and elbow) with limited accuracy.

Furthermore, this skeleton is a planar representation of the human anatomy, and therefore does not really represent the human skeleton in 3D. It must be stressed that in order to be used in clinics for the evaluation and the follow-up of patients, the standard provided skeleton must be improved to include anatomical knowledge to meet anatomical and clinical conventions. A new Model-Based Approach (MBA) that has been specially developed for Kinect input based on previous validated anatomical and biomechanical studies performed (Sholukha et al. 2013). This approach allows real 3D motion analysis of complex movements respecting conventions expected in biomechanics and clinical motion analysis (Bonnechère et al. 2013).

7.3.2   Telemonitoring

Thanks to the generalization of the use of new technology, there is currently more and more electronic devices (laptops, tablets, smartphone, and smartwatch) installed at home. All these devices could be used to monitor people (motions tracking, monitor the mental health, cardiac functions, food intake, etc.).

Since the hardware is, most of the time, already at home, effort must be done on the development of new software.

For example, the project TEKI[3] has been developed for telemonitoring of patients with mental disorders. TEKI proposes a change in the doctor–patient relationship paradigm making easier the use of technology for people with low level of education and/or cognitive impairment.

We have already seen that the risk of fall is one of the most problematic situations for elderly people because it induces lots of adverse effects and comorbidities in case of fractures. Solutions have been developed to use the Kinect sensors as a tool to evaluate the risk of fall and detect people that are most likely to fall. Different kinds of solutions have been proposed: automated test and evaluation during medical consultation (Colagiorgio et al. 2014) or telemonitoring at home to evaluate the patients continuously (Rantz et al. 2015).

In the future, we could also use the motions performed in the serious games to monitor patients and detect if something got wrong during the treatment (Bonnechère et al. 2017).

7.3.3 Evaluation of Clinical Trial

Serious games could be used to monitor the patients during clinical trials. Different approaches can be considered (Byrom 2015).

The first one is directly linked to the functional evaluation: the games could be used to measure objective health outcomes with more sensitivity than the scales and scores currently used to assess patient.

Another approach is to use the games to drive positive patients' compliance behavior and reduce unnecessary withdrawals during clinical studies (e.g., the game Re-Mission designed to increase the compliance to treatment for children with cancer).

The last approach is to educate patients about clinical trial to encourage consideration of trial participation and adherence to treatment.

7.3.4 Haptic and Robotic Devices

Different techniques and approaches of the telerehabilitation have been presented in this book. We were mainly focusing on the use of commercial video games or the use of specially developed games for rehabilitation (using the hardware developed for commercial games). There is one important aspect of the use of new technology in rehabilitation that we do not have addressed: the use of haptic devices.

The haptic sense recreates the sense of touch by applying force, vibrations, or motions to the user[4].

---

[3] http://ec.europa.eu/digital-agenda/events/cf/psp0113-ob3/item-display.cfm?id=10152.
[4] http://www.isfh.org/ch.html.

The use of robot is quite popular in neurologic rehabilitation to help the motion, to provide a feedback to the user, to create vibration during the motion, to provide resistance to motion, etc.

The most known, and oldest example, of this kind of equipment is the passive knee rehabilitation device: a system designed for early rehabilitation after total knee replacement. This device performs flexion-extension movements of the knee to avoid muscle contraction and regain a functional range of motion.

This "robot" is quite rudimentary since it allows only one degree of freedom and does not adjust the amplitude or the force to the patients, those factors must be adjusted by the physiotherapist.

Currently, two main types of robots are being developed for physical rehabilitation: system for gait rehabilitation and systems designed for the upper limbs.

Before robotic gait rehabilitation system, rehabilitation of a patient with spinal cord injury required three clinicians: one to stabilize the trunk and two to mobilize the lower limbs in order to reproduce the gait. Two major problems were related to this technique: the cost since three therapists must be present during the session and the discomfort of the therapists who had to be kneeled to move the patients' legs! Therefore, robots that support patients and assist them to perform the motion, fully supported and doing all the motions in the beginning before gradually becoming more and more passive, is a valuable tool for the rehabilitation of patients suffering from various neurological disorders. These devices (e.g., Lokomat) can also be combined with virtual reality systems or serious games to perform dual-task training and increase the benefit of the rehabilitation.

The other important field of robotics rehabilitation is upper limbs rehabilitation.

Different options are possible depending on the capacity of the patients from relatively simple systems allowing two degrees of freedom: most often a table equipped with a robotic arm that guides the movements of the patient to gradually move towards more functional and complex systems with six degrees of freedom able to reproduce all the complex 3D motions of the upper limbs.

One of the biggest advantages of robotics rehabilitation is the adjustment of the force exerted by the device according to the force generated by the patient. Robotic devices can be used to fully perform the motion or can be used to create resistance or to slow down the motion. These systems can also induce disturbances, forces, or motions that will reinforce the learning and the rehabilitation.

7.3.5 Orthosis

Orthosis are external devices used to support and assist the motion of one or multiple joints. There are static orthosis used to lock and protect the joint and dynamic orthosis that allow some motions. If static devices have been used for hundreds of years (splints created with a branch used to stabilize a bone or joint), dynamic devices are newer. Currently active and dynamic devices not only supporting the joint but also allowing some motions are being developed and tested with patients.

Prostheses are systems that replace limbs. As with orthosis, there is a new paradigm between totally passive systems used for years and increasingly active and intelligent systems currently developed that allow patients to perform more functional and complex motions.

7.3.6 Virtual Reality

Virtual reality is composed of different disciplines: augmented reality, substituted reality, mixed reality, etc.

The aim of virtual reality is to recreate artificially an environment—visual, olfactory, audio, tactile—to immerse the subjects or the patient. The augmented reality is the addition of new information that overlays information from the real world. The substituted reality is the opposite way: The goal is to subtract real information from the real environment, to do so a camera records what the subject is seeing, and to project this information on a virtual reality device. Then, it is possible to modify the reality according to the needs and specificities of the rehabilitation program or the games.

The goal of virtual reality is to dupe the brain by creating an inadequacy between visual, tactile, auditory perceptions, and the reality. The advantage of this immersion in the virtual world is that a multitude of situations can be easily recreated that place the patient in various situations compared to the traditional rehabilitation session. Different regions of the brain can be stimulated and a faster and/or more optimal recovery of those functions can thus be achieved.

This therapeutic principle is of course not, totally, innovative for rehabilitation since it is the same principle used in the mirror therapy (Altschuler et al. 1999).

7.3.7 Machine Learning and Artificial Intelligence

We discussed about telemonitoring and the different kind of devices used for telerehabilitation. In a more general context, the sensors are everywhere: around us (cameras in the street, thermal control camera in the airport), at home (motion analyzer to prevent risk of fall), on the body (watch with heart rate monitor, smartphone with pedometer), and even inside the body (biosensors, prosthesis). All these sensors collect a huge amount of data.

In order to get relevant and useful information from this huge dataset, machine learning algorithms have been developed. These algorithms are designed to find similar profiles in databases by comparing a large sample of data (variables). It is then relatively easy to predict the behavior of an individual by analyzing the behavior of many other users close to this subject.

In the medical field, such techniques are used to try to adapt the treatment and intervention of the patients.

The role of the clinicians is to choose the best type of treatment for each patient based of the clinical history, the environmental factors, etc. is the role of the clinician. Currently, those decisions are based on the medical background but also on the experience, developed with practice, and sometimes on intuition and feeling.

Tomorrow theses decisions must be taken with the support of the technology. The final decision must, of course, be taken by the clinicians but data mining and other techniques should be used of facilitate the diagnosis and increase the quality of the treatment.

References

Altschuler EL, Wisdom SB, Stone L, Foster C, Galasko D, Llewellyn DM, Ramachandran VS. Rehabilitation of hemiparesis after stroke with a mirror. Lancet. 1999;353(9169):2035–6.

Bonnechère B, Sholukha V, Moiseev F, Rooze M, Van Sint Jan S. Patient follow-up using serious games. In: Schouten B, Fedtke S, Bekker T, Schijven M, Gekker A, editors. From Kinect™ to anatomically-correct motion modelling: preliminary results for human application. Wiesbaden: Springer; 2013. p. 15–26.

Bonnechère B, Jansen B, Salvia P, Bouzahouene H, Omelina L, Moiseev F, Sholukha V, Cornelis J, Rooze M, Van Sint Jan S. Validity and reliability of the Kinect within functional assessment activities: comparison with standard stereophotogrammetry. Gait Posture. 2014a;39(1):593–8.

Bonnechère B, Sholukha V, Jansen B, Omelina L, Rooze M, Van Sint Jan S. Determination of repeatability of kinect sensor. Telemed J E Health. 2014b;20(5):451–3.

Bonnechère B, Jansen B, Van Sint Jan S. Cost-effective (gaming) motion and balance deveices for functional assessment: need or hype? J Biomech. 2016;49(13):2561–5.

Bonnechère B, Jansen B, Omelina L, Sholukha V, Van Sint Jan S. Patients' follow-up using bio-mechanial analysis of rehabilitation exercises. Int J Serious Games. 2017;4(1):3–13.

Byrom B. Clinical trials re-spec: the role of games and gamification in the future of clinical trials. In: International Conference on Interactive Technologies and Games (iTAG), 2015.

Cippitelli E, Gasparrini S, Spinsante S, Gambi E. Kinect as a tool for gait analysis: validation of a real-time joint extraction algorithm working in side view. Sensors (Basel). 2015;15(1):1417–34.

Clark RA, Bryant AL, Pua Y, McCrory P, Bennell K, Hunt M. Validity and reliability of the Nintendo Wii balance board for assessment of standing balance. Gait Posture. 2010;31(3):307–10.

Colagiorgio P, Romano F, Sardi F, Moraschini M, Sozzi A, Bejor M, Ricevuti G, Buizza A, Ramat S. Affordable, automatic quantitative fall risk assessment based on clinical balance scales and Kinect data. Conf Proc IEEE Eng Med Biol Soc. 2014;2014:3500–3.

Huurnink A, Fransz DP, Kingma I, van Dieën JH. Comparison of a laboratory grade force platform with a Nintendo Wii balance board on measurement of postural control in single-leg stance balance tasks. J Biomech. 2013;46(7):1392–5.

Laver K, Ratcliffe J, George S, Burgess L, Crotty M. Is the Nintendo Wii fit really acceptable to older people? A discrete choice experiment. BMC Geriatr. 2011;11:64.

Nirme J, Duff A, Verschure PF. Adaptive rehabilitation gaming system: on-line individualization of stroke rehabilitation. Conf Proc IEEE Eng Med Biol Soc. 2011;2011:6749–52.

Omelina L, Jansen B, Bonnechère B, Van Sint Jan S, Cornelis J. Serious games for physical reha-bilitation: designing highly configurable and adaptable games. In: ICDVRAT, Laval, France; 2012.

Perez S, Benitez R, Reinkensmeyer DJ. Smart calibration for video game play by people with a movement impairment. Conf Proc IEEE Eng Med Biol Soc. 2011;2011:6741–4.

Plow M, Finlayson M. A qualitative study exploring the usability of Nintendo Wii fit among per-sons with multiple sclerosis. Occup Ther Int. 2014;21(1):21–32.

Prensky M. Digital game-based learning: practical ideas for the applications of digital game-based learning. St-Paul: Paragon House; 2007.

Rantz M, Skubic M, Abbott C, Galambos C, Popescu M, Keller J, Stone E, Back J, Miller SJ, Petroski GF. Automated in-home fall risk assessment and detection sensor system for elders. Gerontologist. 2015;55(S1):S78–87.

Sholukha V, Bonnechère B, Salvia P, Moiseev F, Rooze M, Van Sint Jan S. Model-based approach for human kinematics reconstruction from markerless and marker-based motion analysis sys-tem. J Biomech. 2013;46(14):2563–71.

Conclusion

The aim of this book was to give an overview of the current use of serious games in physical rehabilitation by presenting the available technology and the status of the clinical validation of this kind of intervention.

The main question was to determine if serious games can be used, and be efficient, in physical rehabilitation. This is obviously not a yes or no question but several points related to this new trend of rehabilitation were addressed: the technological issues, the rehabilitation point of view, and several problems that still need to be fixed.

Therefore, we hope that after reading this book the reader has a more precise idea and opinion about the possibilities offered by the serious games, but also the limitations.

We have seen that, thanks to the development of new technology and the gaming industry, more and more sophisticated solutions are being developed and are available for patients.

Currently the general trend is, still, that the devices used in clinics are first developed for gaming purpose only—the gaming market is much larger and lucrative than the rehabilitation one—such solutions are then adapted and transformed for rehabilitation purposes or used directly with the patients.

In some cases, the games are not adapted at all for patients and rehabilitation (i.e., visual complexity, motions, speed) but the gaming devices could be used for rehabilitation purpose (e.g., Kinect sensor and Wii Balance Board).

We have seen that, slowly but surely, the use of serious games started to emerge in hospital and private practice. Solutions are being developed for the management of various pathologies and therefore the number of patients that could potentially benefit from this kind of intervention is growing and the scientific evidences supporting this intervention are being published.

Some potential investors and entrepreneurs did not miss these opportunities and believe in the future and the development of this field in the health care sector. Companies are created and proposed several applications for telemedicine, telemonitoring, telecare, and telerehabiliation.

Those companies developed and proposed their solutions in a context of uncertainty in terms of legality, safety, and reimboursement. This particular context does not encourage enough new development and there is still not enough investment in this field.

© Springer International Publishing AG 2018
B. Bonnechère, *Serious Games in Physical Rehabilitation*,
https://doi.org/10.1007/978-3-319-66122-3

The three most important factors hampering future development are: safety and responsibility, price and reimboursement, and the state of mind of the users.

The question of the responsibility in case of accident should be discussed at worldwide level no only for serious games but in the global context of the use of new technology and robotics in the health care sector. The legislation is currently far away compared to the development of technology, and there is a huge gap between research and development and the use in daily clinic.

The question about price and reimbursement should also be discussed at higher level in order to prevent medical shopping and to avoid a gap between developed and emerging countries.

The last point is the state of mind. Despite the published studies, a lot of people are still reluctant to use, or even to discuss about, serious games to treat patients. For lots of people, the serious games are still just games and games cannot be used for medical purposes.

Therefore, there is still lot of works to be done in order to continue the development of adapted solutions based on the specificity and need of the rehabilitation scheme and the validation of these solutions by performing a large-scale randomized and controlled clinical trial using the serious games in order to change people's mind and to convince them that serious games are serious and can be used safely to help patients!